Green Babies, Sage Moms

Green Babies, Sage Moms

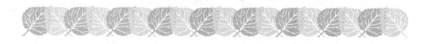

*The Ultimate Guide
to Raising Your
Organic Baby*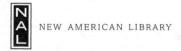

Lynda Fassa

NAL

NEW AMERICAN LIBRARY

New American Library
Published by New American Library, a division of
Penguin Group (USA) Inc., 375 Hudson Street,
New York, New York 10014, USA
Penguin Group (Canada), 90 Eglinton Avenue East, Suite 700, Toronto,
Ontario M4P 2Y3, Canada (a division of Pearson Penguin Canada Inc.)
Penguin Books Ltd., 80 Strand, London WC2R 0RL, England
Penguin Ireland, 25 St. Stephen's Green, Dublin 2,
Ireland (a division of Penguin Books Ltd.)
Penguin Group (Australia), 250 Camberwell Road, Camberwell, Victoria 3124,
Australia (a division of Pearson Australia Group Pty. Ltd.)
Penguin Books India Pvt. Ltd., 11 Community Centre, Panchsheel Park,
New Delhi - 110 017, India
Penguin Group (NZ), 67 Apollo Drive, Rosedale, North Shore 0632,
New Zealand (a division of Pearson New Zealand Ltd.)
Penguin Books (South Africa) (Pty.) Ltd., 24 Sturdee Avenue,
Rosebank, Johannesburg 2196, South Africa

Penguin Books Ltd., Registered Offices: 80 Strand, London WC2R 0RL, England

First published by New American Library, a division of Penguin Group (USA) Inc.

First Printing, January 2008
5 7 9 10 8 6 4

This book is printed on acid-free, recycled paper.

Copyright © Lynda Fassa, 2008
All rights reserved

Green Babies is a trademark of Green Babies, Inc.

REGISTERED TRADEMARK—MARCA REGISTRADA

Library of Congress Cataloging-in-Publication Data
Fassa, Lynda.
Green babies, sage moms : the ultimate guide to raising your organic baby / Lynda Fassa.
p. cm.
ISBN: 978-0-451-22289-3
1. Organic living.   2. Infants—Care.   I. Title.
GF77.F37 2008
649'.1—dc22   2007025728

Set in Adobe Garamond
Designed by Jessica Shatan Heslin/Studio Shatan, Inc.

Printed in the United States of America

PUBLISHER'S NOTE

Every effort has been made to ensure that the information contained in this book is complete and accurate. However, neither the publisher nor the author is engaged in rendering professional advice or services to the individual reader. The ideas, procedures, and suggestions contained in this book are not intended as a substitute for consulting with your physician. All matters regarding your child's health require medical supervision. Neither the author nor the publisher shall be liable or responsible for any loss or damage allegedly arising from any information or suggestion in this book. The opinions expressed in this book represent the personal views of the author and not of the publisher.

The publisher does not have any control over and does not assume any responsibility for author or third-party Web sites or their content.

Acknowledgments

I would like to gratefully acknowledge my agents at William Morris, Brian Dubin, Mel Berger, and Strand Conover, who saw early on how valuable "green" information is to the health and well-being of our children and, indeed, to all of us as a society. I'd also like to say I am the luckiest person in the world to have the love and support of everyone who helped on this project, including my fab sister Dawn Bridges, the gorgeous and witty Krista Smith, the inspirational and enlightened Vanessa Williams, the beautiful super-brain (my best friend) Dr. Lisa Ecklund-Flores, and the smartest voice in my head, my kind and gentle editor, Tracy Bernstein.

But most of all, I want to acknowledge *you*—you parents and caregivers, friends and relatives, who are the gatekeepers and the guardians at the door to protect our most precious and valuable resources, our wonderful and adored children.

Contents

Green Is Good

"The point is, ladies and gentlemen, that green—for lack of a better word—is good. Green is right. Green works.

"Green clarifies, cuts through, and captures the essence of the evolutionary spirit.

"Green, in all of its forms—green for life, for money, for love—has marked the upward surge of mankind."

Well, OK, I did change a letter in one word from that famous speech by Michael Douglas' character in *Wall Street*. But that was then and this is now, and no one can deny the surge in interest in all things environmental. In a world of unfulfilled promises and empty brands, green is the new gold—green matters. Green is on the horizon, organically growing, exponentially expanding into every sector of our lives like Jack's magic beanstalk.

But what does that mean for you, and for your baby?

Green is safe, green is clean, and mothers have an especially vested interest in a toxin-free environment. It is our joy and our job to keep our children safe. After accidents, cancer is the biggest killer of American children. New studies link exposure to household toxins from cleaning products and decor such as vinyl flooring and synthetic carpets not only to cancer but to the growing spike in asthma and even learning disabilities like ADD and ADHD.

There is a better way, a greener way. And before you start to feel even the tiniest bit overwhelmed, understand this: You don't need to move to Montana or be a Una-mommer to get the best alternatives for your baby. (Although Montana is very nice, I hear.)

All you need to do to make the kind of changes that will improve your family's personal environment, your home, and your life is to start with baby steps. Before you know it, you will have taken one giant step for mankind. I'm going to tell you about easy, fun, makes-sense things you can do for yourself and your baby to ensure a happier world where you can feel terrific about going "au naturel."

I am not here to scare you or guilt-trip you. This is a guide to empower you to make informed decisions without completely overhauling your lifestyle or your bank account. At the end of every chapter I'll list changes you can make by their shade of green— from evergreen to pea green to spring green—so whether you're a Birkenstock-wearing tree hugger or somewhat reluctant to part with your SUV, you will choose the level that's right for you.

In addition, I've interviewed the smartest Green Gurus around, a whole passel of world-renowned sages. Throughout the book you'll find their cool, easy—and inexpensive—tips and recipes on how to get "down to earth." I want to share what I've learned to help you with the most important person in the world, your baby.

Thank you so much for including me in this fantastic time in your life. Because of you, it's a whole new world out there—you are literally building your child's tomorrow today. Thanks for helping make it a green one.

¡Viva el verde!
Lynda

Foreword

Congratulations!

If you are reading this book, it means that you or someone you really care about is pregnant or has recently become a member of one of Mother Earth's oldest clubs . . . *PARENTHOOD*.

This club has great perks! The wonderful smell of your baby's hair, the indescribably delicious feeling of that warm cheek pressing softly on yours, the tender innocence of your child asleep in the crib.

But (and this is an important but) the group you have just joined is very much a *dues-paying* club. You'll have to give of yourself . . . big-time: in sleep, stained clothing, missed parties, worry wrinkles, depleted savings, and daily efforts to protect your child from harm.

Recently, protecting our kids from harm required a new type of effort—protecting them from chemicals. That's because we discovered that somewhere back in the 1950s we made a really bad decision. Back then, chemicals were universally applauded as mankind's salvation. We naively believed that our bodies were so strong and the world was so huge that we could release vast—I mean really vast—amounts of toxic and untested chemicals into our air, water, and cities . . . without so much as an "Oops."

Well, we were wrong.

Inevitably, this chemical carnival overwhelmed nature's ability to forgive. Our folly has battered the planet and resulted in today's many environmental crises, like a huge rip in the ozone layer, ocean sectors devoid of fish, and of course global warming.

Our naïveté has also hurt people. The negligent release of tons upon tons of asbestos, lead, pesticides, solvents, and hundreds of other rogue chemicals has caused much sickness and pain.

We clearly have our work cut out for us. And this is where the *dues* part of being a member of the Parenthood Club comes in.

In addition to performing the big job of raising a child, each new wave of parents is called upon to make a larger sacrifice to help its children. Past generations made generous investments in bridges, tunnels, schools, highways, and airports. These are all a gift from them to us.

What gifts will *we* leave to our children? How will the newest generation of parents step up and make a difference? We cannot ignore or evade our obligations. They will only fall on the shoulders of our children and at a much steeper price.

And that's where Lynda Fassa's great book *Green Babies* makes such a contribution.

Green Babies is chock-full of facts, hope, and a smorgasbord of clever ideas to keep your child healthy and happy and to help inspire you to make a difference in your life and the world.

Lynda is right on the money when she points out that today's parents are wiser and more informed than ever before. And we are blessed with an abundance of products that offer us healthy, *green* options. All we have to do is . . . take them home . . . and put them to use.

Now, it's *our* turn to pay the dues.

I have total faith that if we think clearly and pitch in together, we can give our children the gift of a safer, healthier, truly better world. A world they deserve.

Let's start today!

—Dr. Harvey Karp,
author of *The Happiest Baby on the Block*
and *The Happiest Toddler on the Block*

Introduction

How My Green Light Turned On

I started my business, Green Babies, right after my first daughter, Layla, was born, more than thirteen years ago. Today, Green Babies offers the largest selection of organic-cotton clothes for babies and kids on the planet. I've been called a trailblazer and a pioneer in this rapidly exploding industry. But I am really just a mom who had an idea of how I wanted things to be for my baby, and who also needed a job.

Here's how it happened: Layla was a very colicky baby, crying for hours at a time, and that shifted me, pretty quickly, into new priorities. My swanky Peg Perego pram sat unused in the corner. I had imagined escaping my confining city apartment and taking leisurely strolls with my beautiful baby through Washington Square Park in New York City. In reality, I ended up hauling Layla in whatever sling, Snugli, or BabyBjörn seemed to calm her for a few minutes. Honestly, I had thought becoming a mom wouldn't change me. I would just be "the same old Lynda" except now I would occasionally be holding, rocking, or feeding this supercute baby. It would be all about the fun stuff I could do with baby and how nice to have everyone else notice how adorable and cuddly she was, too. This was a vague fantasy, but a very pleasant one.

Until Layla was born, I didn't understand that it wasn't about me anymore—it was about her. Not in a weird slave/washerwoman way, but in a life-affirming, mind-expanding "Who knew life could be so wonderful and fulfilling?" way. Love is a great motivator, one that began the greening of me—and my baby. I had already done a major lifestyle change when I found out I was pregnant—gone were the days of Diet Coke and skipped lunches, replaced by leafy veggies and organic smoothies. Starvation diets and synthetic sweeteners might have been good enough for me (and a necessity during my days as a working model), but they were not good enough for my future baby. Why shouldn't she have the very best of everything I could provide? More complicated choices, but equally important ones, had to be made after she was born. I loved this baby intensely, with my whole heart, but parenting her was very different from how I thought it would be, and would require me to make some major adjustments on my part for me to step up to my new role as her mother. (They actually need to eat—several times a day! And, no, you can't just pop out for a spontaneous dinner with your mate and leave baby for an hour or two, the way I did with our friendly shelter mutt.)

On top of that, I needed a new job. My baby weight—an extra twenty pounds—made modeling in New York impossible. I wondered what I could possibly do with my limited education. Then I read a story in the *New York Times* about Texas cotton farmers abandoning their pesticide-based way of agriculture and returning to a more natural way, what we now call organic. I learned cotton is the second-most pesticide-laden crop in the world, and number one in America. It takes up only three percent of the world's farmland but uses twenty-five percent of the world's chemical pesticides and fertilizers! Now, remember, I was under the "estrogen veil"—i.e., very weepy and emotional—and I cried as I read how these noble, salt-of-the-earth farmers were risking everything, giving up federal subsidies and losing bank loans, to make safer, toxin-free choices for the rest of us. They saw what we couldn't see from our city lofts and suburban backyards. They knew that what killed the pests, dropped from planes flying high above, also landed in unpredictable places and killed much else, as well.

I loved this story, and I knew something about fashion from my years modeling Jean Paul Gaultier and Karl Lagerfeld. So I decided to make baby clothes from organic cotton and started Green Babies out of my apartment, with a lot of hope and a few credit cards.

Since those exhilarating first days, I have had the pleasure of speaking with thousands of new mothers, and I know for sure that we are all sisters, that regardless of the many differences between us, we share one powerful, unbreakable bond. Our children bring all kinds of wonderful gifts with them when they enter the world, and offer us an opportunity—a challenge, really—to grow, change, and improve. (When my first child was born, she brought me a whole new perspective on everything from my lack of foresight as to how many diapers we'd need for an afternoon on the town—at least eight—to the true nature of reality and my place in it—haven't figured that one out yet!)

Even though my kids are now fourteen, eleven, and eight, I know there's no done deal with parenting—and no one right answer. But I do firmly believe that natural is better. I believe we have a responsibility to do the best we can for our kids. We, as a culture, have been putting our most valuable and vulnerable resources—our children—at needless risk of birth defects, learning disabilities, asthma, and even cancer, sometimes just by the products we use every day. In this book I want to share with you the simple things that you can do to reduce your and your family's exposure to toxins. There are loads of ways you can make the world a better place for your child, and for children everywhere, and some don't even cost a cent.

So read on, friend, sister, mother (and dad!), and take what feels right for you. (And to that other little person who can't read yet—welcome to the world, baby—we love you!)

"What joy is welcomed like a newborn child?"

—DOROTHY L. NOLTE

Part I

Pregnancy: A Green Pea in the Pod

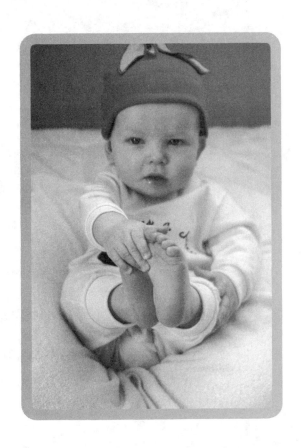

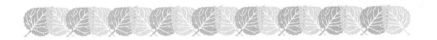

Congratulations! You are expecting a baby and your baby is going to be wonderful. It really is the most fun you'll ever have in your life. I know, sometimes it's hard to feel that way in the beginning. The first four months of pregnancy are incredibly important but are usually the most difficult for the mother. Maybe you feel fat. Your breasts may be sore. You may have strange cravings or be hit by waves of nausea that can range from a ripple to a tidal wave. You may feel panicked about what you put in your mouth and what you put on your skin and what they are doing to the baby growing inside you. Worse yet, perhaps you don't want to tell anyone because you could still lose the pregnancy, yet you need to make changes in your lifestyle.

We've all heard of things to avoid during pregnancy such as smoking (well, not just during pregnancy!), caffeine, soft cheeses, and sushi. But there's more to it than that. What can be safe for the mother can be incredibly toxic for a fetus (no more trips to Margaritaville, at least for the time being). Then there are things that are not good for either of you at any time, such as volatile organic compounds. You're surrounded by VOCs, a class of solvents lurking everywhere, even in some prized personal-care items like nail polishes and removers and certain hair products.

You also really want to steer clear of things that are developed to kill, pesticides. In this first section we'll cover organic foods—why you need them and how to choose the most important ones to reduce your, and your baby's, exposure to pesticides. We'll also look into the body beautiful. Your changing body is your baby's first home, and we'll explore how what you put *on* your body may be as important to your baby's health as what you put *in* your body.

Then we'll tackle housekeeping. The nesting urge strikes most pregnant women (even me!), often toward the end of our pregnancies, and even "relaxed" housekeepers can become driven Domestic Divas. However, many of the ingredients in regular household cleaning supplies are questionable, even dangerous. I'll help you put together a cleaning regimen that's really clean and green.

There's also my favorite chapter in the section: ideas for the baby party of the year, a green baby shower! One even Mother Nature would be proud of! Woo-hoo, welcome, baby! Now, on to the good work of helping build the healthiest and happiest green baby you can!

One 🍃
Food for Thought

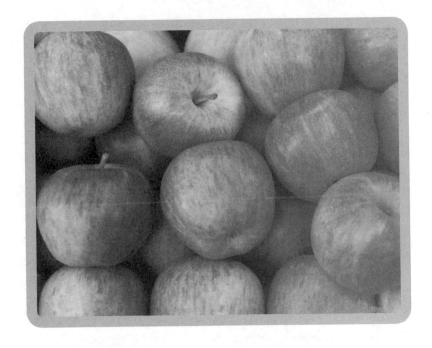

You Are What You Eat— and So Is Your Baby

Y ou need an extra 750 calories a day when you're expecting. Sounds fun—and it is, but not all calories are created equal. You are a glowing baby factory, and what you choose to consume will never be more important. Everything that you put into your mouth (especially in the first trimester) is the stuff you are using to build your baby. Generally speaking, the fresher the food you eat, and the closer to its natural state, the greater its nutritional value—more bang for the caloric buck. Although there's nothing wrong with stashing an occasional energy bar in your bag to equalize your blood sugar roller coaster, a banana or an apple is even better.

You may occasionally slip and inhale a bag of salty potato chips, but probably you've already committed to a fresh and healthy diet for baby's sake. But what is healthy, really, and what about all the hoopla regarding organic food? Is organic really better for you, and your beautiful bump? Or just a gimmick, and an expensive one at that?

People often ask me: What is "organic"? There is a host of very specific and wonderful things that define "organic," but most importantly and simply put, here is what organic means:

Produced without pesticides, because pesticides are poison.

Consider this: The Environmental Protection Agency (EPA) states, "There is no safe level of pesticides, only those with an acceptable level of risk."

But when what you eat is forming the most important person in the world, that doesn't sound so "acceptable."

How did this "risk" become such a huge part of our food chain? Do we need pesticides to grow food? It seems almost unbelievable that we have come to a point where we are risking our health, individually and as a society—including the health of people we absolutely depend on to survive in this world, farmers—because of a food system that depends on poison to work.

Conventional agriculture in America is subsidized by the federal government. Often farmers are paid to NOT grow crops so that the super-low prices of the subsidized goods don't go even lower. In the late 1940s, after the Second World War, American industry was booming. Many of the chemicals that had been developed for the war were still in high production. It was discovered that the poisons developed during the war to combat the gargantuan mosquitoes of North Africa and Southeast Asia could be used against another threat, crop-eating bugs.

This simple idea became linked to the promise of bounty for all, an effortless end to shortage and starvation. At the outset this seemed like a potentially beautiful solution—chemistry could liberate us from toil and provide an endless abundance. What went wrong? It is still possible chemistry will provide that Utopia, but at the moment we are looking at a much darker picture.

True, we *produce* more than enough for all, but things are out of whack—there is still rampant malnutrition and even starvation. Cheap food became a boon for affluent consumers, but a bane for farmers. Industrial agriculture and its super-high yields demand more and more chemicals, and push the land so hard that we have wiped out entire ecosystems. Farms, once living landscapes filled with rich biological variety, have become arid wastelands that produce flavorless food and poison surrounding communities and waterways with their chemical runoff, in much the same way the manufacturing industry did a hundred years ago. Chemically dependent agriculture has also brought us epic deforestation, rising cancer rates, an end to the era of the family farm, and a business climate that sees over thirty thousand suicides by farmers annually, many related to debt to chemical companies. Can we really continue to drop poison—poison strong enough to kill resistant insects—on our food supply and think everything will be OK?

GOT FAT?

And there are other risks with conventional farming. Scientists have speculated that the rise in obesity in the West is connected to the growth hormones and genetic engineering inflicted on the American dairy cow. If we (and our children) consume milk from cows that are goaded into growing abnormally large and producing so much more than is natural for them, it is possible that what made those cows so big and fat might do the same to us. We simply do not know how years of consuming rBGH milk and dairy products will affect our health. But we do know that rBGH, or bovine growth hormone, is administered to cows so they produce more milk, and antibiotics are then given to treat and reduce the sometimes resulting infections—infections that can have extremely unpleasant results, such as pus in the milk—so you may be getting a dose of tetracycline in your latte. If that doesn't convince you, some studies suggest a link between cancer and rBGH. According to Dr. Samuel Epstein of the University of Illinois at Chicago, "GE [genetically engineered] milk is entirely different from natural milk: nutritionally; biochemically; and immunologically. It is also contaminated with antibiotics used to treat mastitis and pus; the GE hormone; and high levels of the naturally occurring growth factor IGF-1. Elevated levels of IGF-1 have been strongly associated with high risk of colon, breast and prostate cancers, besides promoting their invasiveness. In spite of such well-documented scientific evidence, FDA approved the sales and marketing of GE milk in 1984, while blocking all labeling" (Samuel Epstein, MD, "Statement on Public Health Hazards of GE Milk and Food"). Dr. Epstein further says, "With the active complicity of the FDA, the entire nation is currently being subjected to an experiment involving large-scale adulteration of an age-old dietary staple by a poorly characterized and unlabeled biotechnology product, BGH [biosynthetic growth hormones], which is genetically engineered by Monsanto. Even more disturbingly, it poses major potential health risks for the entire U.S. population" (Epstein, "Unlabeled Milk from Cows Treated with Biosynthetic Growth Hormones: A Case of Regulatory Abdication," *International Journal of Health Services* 26, no. 1, 1996: 173–85).

The Food and Drug Administration (FDA), unlike the government in other nations, has sided with the manufacturer of rBGH (Monsanto) and decided U.S. consumers do not need to know which dairy products have been produced with rBGH, so there is no label you can check. However, by choosing organic milk, you don't have to guess. Organic milk means no rBGH, no synthetic hormones, and no antibiotics are given to the dairy cows producing the milk.

GROWING GREEN

When you're expecting, organic makes sense for fruits and vege-tables and grain, too. Conventional produce grown with heavy doses of pesticides developed to kill hardy insects, and dropped from planes flying high above onto the food we eat, is not the best choice, especially when you're in baby-factory mode. If there was a fly on your apple, would you spray it with Raid, wash it off, and eat it? Sounds ridiculous, but it's basically what we're doing every day. Worst of all, we are doing it to foods that are otherwise especially life-giving and healthy—fresh fruits and vegetables. And these pesticides don't just contaminate our produce. They harm our water quality in a number of different ways. They seep into groundwater on the farm, and also go back into the eco-system as we work to wash them down the drain in our kitchen sinks.

How can you reduce your and your unborn baby's exposure to these health risks? The shining ray of hope and health is organics.

In order for foods to be certified organic they must meet a se-ries of strict criteria, including that

- no synthetic pesticides, fertilizers, or herbicides were used on the crop (or land) for at least three years;

- there are no GMOs (genetically modified organisms);

- in the case of meat and dairy, no growth hormones or anti-biotics were given to the animals and all feed was vegetarian and certified organic.

Red Flag

Here are the Dirty Dozen—the conventionally grown foods you most want to avoid because of their high rates of pesticides:

apples	peaches
bell peppers	pears
celery	potatoes
cherries	red raspberries
imported grapes	spinach
nectarines	strawberries

Green Flag

Here are the Tempting Twelve—healthful and delicious fruits and veggies that, even when grown conventionally, expose you to fairly low amounts of pesticides:

asparagus	kiwis
avocados	mangoes
bananas	onions
broccoli	papaya
cauliflower	peas
corn	pineapples

Keep in mind, though, that any conventionally grown food you buy was grown with pesticides, and even if you personally are not consuming much of their residues, like in the case of bananas, the toxins are still in the environment and will have an effect not only on whoever is involved in the growing process but on the land somewhere. By choosing organic, you are supporting a cleaner and more sustainable world.

Green Guru

Janelle Hope Robbins
STAFF SCIENTIST, WATERKEEPER ALLIANCE

There are some really, really smart people who devote themselves to making life better for all of us. People who turn their brilliant minds to books and studies, not simply for the joy of learning, but to help us in the challenges we've created here on the planet. Janelle Hope Robbins is one of these people, working to ensure your kids are not swimming in PCBs or drinking water filled with lead. Of all the great gifts we enjoy on earth, none are as intimately tied to our health and well-being as water. Waterkeeper Alliance is a grassroots advocacy organization—with 157 local programs and growing—dedicated to preserving and protecting our water from polluters.

"It's always best to choose organic. Organic produce is grown without harmful pesticides and sewage sludge.

"Some people say that if you're peeling the food, it doesn't matter whether you buy organic. Yes, the peel gets thrown away, after the pesticides applied to the crops have already drifted into neighbors' yards and homes, seeped into groundwater and drinking-water wells, and run off into streams and rivers—polluting habitat- and drinking-water sources. The peel gets thrown away after the pesticide has poisoned both pests and wildlife, after it has been inhaled and ingested by farmworkers, and after you have brought the poison into your vehicles and your homes. The peel gets thrown away long after the pesticides have gotten on your kids' hands. The EPA and USDA say these poisons are safe, but how much poison is really safe?

"Is organic expensive? You get what you pay for. Say you're comparing the price of Organic Valley milk to the price of conventional store-brand milk. You may think to yourself, 'Is a glass of organic milk worth X more than conventional milk?' However, Organic Valley is more than just a supplier of organic products; it is a cooperative of organic family farms across the nation. Organic Valley is instrumental in preserving the family-farm way of life, which is threatened by industrial agriculture. Industrial agriculture pollutes our soil, air, and water; alienates farmworkers and neighbors; destroys rural communities; and puts family farms out of business—all to make the biggest profit possible. So while the higher price of Organic Valley products stems partially from the higher cost of organic practices, it is also because they support family farms. With conventional factory farming, consumers are increasingly disconnected from their food: where it comes from, who grows it, and how it ends up on the dinner table. Just because conventional produce, meat, and dairy products don't pose direct or immediate harm to you and your family doesn't mean that they haven't already harmed someone else or that they aren't going to harm you in the future. The bottom line: If you care about the future, buy organic whenever you can."

The good news is that because of skyrocketing consumer demand for all things organic, it is now much easier and less expensive to find organic products. Most large-chain grocery stores carry at least one brand of organic milk and organic eggs. Some even have a lower-priced private-label brand, like Stop & Shop's Nature's Promise. If you're lucky enough to have a Whole Foods Market near you, you'll be able to get the best organic everything! And much of it will come from local farmers, so you'll know your purchases are supporting your local economy and reducing carbon emissions, too.

But it's not just Whole Foods, Mrs. Green's, or the local food co-op anymore. Wal-Mart has now pledged to carry up to two hundred different certified-organic offerings, including cornflakes, ketchup, and chips—yes, chips! Is junk food that's organic better for you? Actually, organic junk food is not an oxymoron. Again, organic means grown without synthetic pesticides—junky food without chemical poisons may not be as healthful as healthy food without poison, but at least it's not adding to your body's chemical burden. In other words, if you really need a cheese puff, it is better to indulge in a bag made from corn grown without pesticides and whose flavorings come from fat, salt, and cheese rather than the chemical burdens of MSG and a host of other synthetic, lab-generated "flavors."

GREEN TO GO It's getting easier to combine the benefits of organic with the luxury of home delivery. Got a craving for grass-fed organic lamb? A fully prepared meal for your in-laws? The most divine organic chocolates? Check out Diamond Organics (www.diamond organics.com). I personally loved the sampler-of-the-month program, a fresh combo of organic foods delivered to you on a regular basis. Plus, when my kids got older they really looked forward to that box arriving and it was a great way for them to try some exotic fruits and veggies. They offer nationwide overnight delivery on most things.

GREEN GRAPES

If you're feeling well enough to entertain (and better to throw that dinner party now, because you'll be even busier when baby's born!), you may want to consider the libations your guests will be enjoying (of course you won't be indulging in any vino right now!). Yep, wine has gone organic, too.

If that sounds funny to you, remember, grapes are one of the most pesticide-laden crops in the world! Up to 240 different chemicals are involved in the making of conventional wines. Conversely, organic wines are made with grapes grown without chemical fertilizers, herbicides, or insecticides that can hurt soil, plants, and wildlife—and ultimately show up in the wine. Instead, biologically active soil is maintained in vineyards through alternatives such as cultivating the soil and planting cover crops, using natural fertilizers, promoting a biodiversity of plants, and encouraging natural predators of insect pests. Also, processing (such as filtration and clarifying) is kept to a minimum, without any chemical additives. Organic wines are produced using minimal sulfites. This ensures great taste and freshness, and prevents oxidation, as winemakers have known for thousands of years. Added bonus? The greatly reduced sulfite content of organic wines means greatly reduced side effects, like fewer hangovers and headaches, for the many people who are sulfite-sensitive.

Ask your local wine store if they carry organics or can get them. Look for news on the benefits of organic wine at www.organicvintners.com. Organic Vintners will also ship their vast variety of certified-organic wines to twenty states in the continental U.S., and they've got it all, even biodynamic and vegan wines.

Green Guru

Dan Barber
CHEF, BLUE HILL AT STONE BARNS

In lower Westchester County sits a bucolic town called Pocantico Hills. Cottages dot the country lanes and cows lazily graze the pastures. But this is no ordinary town. The Rockefeller estate Kykuit hugs the main road and the local church has windows by Chagall and Matisse. As past generations contributed to society through philanthropy and art, the Rockefellers have now turned their eyes to sustainability. On the edge of town is Stone Barns, their working organic farm, where families, school groups, and just the curious can spend a day strolling about or helping with the harvest. At Blue Hill, its restaurant, everything on every plate comes directly from the farm. (Oh, and in case you're thinking "how quaint," you'll be lucky if you can get a reservation even when calling two months ahead!)

"Why does local matter? Health. Taste. Environment. Local is it. Local should rule the day over everything else. Buying direct from a local farmer means produce is picked at the optimal time, when it's had time to mature properly, and delivered straight to you with no storage in between. Tasty vegetables and delicious meats don't happen by accident.

"In some ways, we have reduced the idea of 'organic' to a farming method. But there's much more to it. Who is growing your food? Where is it coming from? What's the carbon footprint? Flying a five-calorie strawberry from California—that's just not environmentally economical. Understand the history on your plate. Shake the hand of the person growing your food.

"If you're bringing someone into the world, you want to think about the world you're constructing. Food is a very powerful vehicle to effect change."

Roasted Fennel with a Salad of Mâche and Pickled Fennel
SERVES 4

2 medium fennel bulbs, trimmed and halved
2 tablespoons olive oil
2 cups mâche
4 tablespoons pickled fennel (recipe to follow)
lemon vinaigrette (recipe to follow)
salt and pepper to taste

1. Preheat oven to 375 degrees.
2. Season fennel with salt and pepper. Add 2 tablespoons of oil to an ovenproof nonstick sauté pan and, over a medium-high heat, sear fennel on cut side for 1 minute. Move sauté pan to oven and continue to cook for 10 minutes or until the fennel is fork tender.
3. To serve, season mâche with salt and pepper, dress with

lemon vinaigrette, and toss in pickled fennel. Plate along-side roasted fennel.

Pickled Fennel

10 heads fennel
1 teaspoon fennel seeds
1 teaspoon black peppercorns
24 ounces rice-wine vinegar
2 tablespoons salt
5 tablespoons sugar
thyme sprigs for garnish (optional)

1. Slice fennel on mandolin.
2. Place fennel seeds and peppercorns in a medium pot and toast lightly over a medium flame.
3. Add vinegar, salt, and sugar and bring to a simmer. Add sliced fennel.
4. Remove from heat, chill, and store in refrigerator.

Lemon Vinaigrette

2 tablespoons Dijon mustard
¼ cup lemon juice
¼ cup lemon oil (recipe below)
¼ cup extra-virgin olive oil (Use really delicious olive oil—it will make a big difference!)

In a medium bowl combine mustard and lemon juice. Slowly whisk in lemon oil and olive oil. Season to taste.

Lemon Oil

1 quart canola oil
4 pieces lemon zest
¼ bunch lemon thyme
¼ stick lemongrass

1. In a medium saucepan combine all ingredients. Place over a very low heat for 1 hour. Do not let oil boil.
2. Remove from heat, cool, and strain. Refrigerate until ready to use.

It's really all about you. You're the boss. The captain of the ship. The one who signs the checks. You have an opportunity to change the world and vote with your wallet. In fact, you and I are doing that every day, whether we are consciously aware of it or not. A friend of mine who's a terrific chef, Katie Lee Joel, introduced me to the concept of *conscious consumption*—how to lead the really good life by enjoying what you eat, buy, and support. As we parents ponder the state of the world we are bringing our babies into, we all want to create positive changes.

The easiest and most effective way to drive positive change is to connect to your own power—to be a conscious consumer: Purchase products and food from businesses whose ideals you trust and want to support. How do they treat their employees? What is their impact in the immediate community? How about the world at large? Wherever you plunk down your cash, you are supporting their way of doing business. Is it business as usual? Or business unusual—a business that is actually making the world better?

Our dollars can make business unusual into the new norm. In fact, it's already started, with many Fortune 500 companies looking to rebrand themselves as green to garner customer loyalty in an increasingly competitive world market.

There are long-term effects to everything that we buy and eat, from how it was produced, to how far it has traveled, to how it was packaged, to the actual store we purchase it in, to how its makers treat their workers, vendors, and communities. We have marvelous choices in everything—more than kings and queens in times past. We are very powerful. Don't think you have to fall into the fear zone, but buy instead out of knowledge and joy. It makes the world seem like a much nicer place, for us and for our children.

GIVING UP THAT FAB FRIEND, CAFFEINE During my first pregnancy, I had no trouble at all giving up coffee—the smell alone sent me running for the bathroom—but that was not true for many of my girlfriends, who found it more difficult to give up a swarthy cup of java than to push their favorite Donna Karan to the back of the closet until the next (skinny) year. Many of those friends had half a cup of java with a lot of milk (with their doctor's OK) or switched to decaf. But all decaf is not created equal, and you might be getting more than you bargained for. (And speaking of which, please, please steer clear of any synthetic sweeteners. Sugar is the only way to go during pregnancy, since even honey can carry potentially dangerous microbes.) Michael Love of Coffee Labs Roasters in Tarrytown, New York, has a huge selection of organic and fair trade coffee, and a lot of it is decaf. "There are different ways to get caffeine out of coffee," says Love, "including with chemicals. Look for coffee that is decaffeinated by a water process, such as Swiss Water. That way when you're chugging a cup of decaf, there're no extra nasty chemicals."

GREEN AT A GLANCE

Evergreen: Know where your food comes from, and how it was grown—even who grew it, if possible (see localharvest.org to look via zip code for local farmers near you).

Pea green: Be a conscious consumer. Ask, do you need this product? And is it high in ethical or nutritional value?

Spring green: Choose organic for the Dirty Dozen. You'll feel good about what you are doing for your family and ensure cleaner drinking water and soil in the agricultural community.

Two

Beauty Is More Than Skin Deep

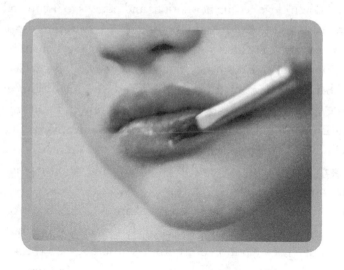

How Cosmetics and Skin-Care Products May Affect Your Developing Baby

Most of us, if given the chance, are product addicts. Who doesn't love getting new lotions and potions to use in and out of the bath and shower? And who doesn't want to diminish those laugh lines and crow's-feet with a promising face or eye cream?

It's no wonder the cosmetics industry is a multibillion-dollar one.

When you are pregnant, cosmetics can be especially appealing. While your waistline is growing and your stomach is churning, a spirit-lifting liquid eyeliner might seem like a great idea. But did you know that the blushes, mascaras, and other prettifiers you are using might actually be toxic to you and could be pure poison to your baby?

Yes, it seems absurd. How can a plain old foundation or lipstick harm a fetus? But the skin is the body's largest organ. Sixty percent of what we put on our bodies is absorbed into the skin. If in doubt, consider the effectiveness of the nicotine patch. The Chinese call the skin the third lung because it is such a direct pathway to our bloodstream!

Toxic beauty products are not new. European aristocrats applied powdered lead to their faces, and Victorian beauties smeared their faces with arsenic-laced creams. We have come a long way, but unfortunately not far enough. The Food and Drug Administration does not oversee the safety of most ingredients in cosmetics. There is no board regulating the amount of toxins—often in the form of preservatives—in our makeup.

And if you think these toxins are present only in cheap products, think again. They are in some of the most expensive and luxurious big-name brands available, the kind you see in swanky department stores and advertised on the pages of glossy magazines.

Warning! Scary Information to Follow

The biggest offenders and most pervasive ingredients are called *parabens* (common examples: methylparaben, propylparaben, ethylparaben, butylparaben). About ninety-nine percent of all consumer cosmetics contain one or more parabens, a group of powerful preservatives that extend a product's shelf life.

• A 2004 British study in *Journal of Applied Toxicology* cited parabens as a "cause for concern." After finding traces of parabens in the tumors of twenty women with breast cancer, the scientists concluded that there is a link between parabens and breast cancer. Studies have linked products containing parabens to a variety of hormone disorders, including underdeveloped testes in infant boys.

• Over and over, parabens have been linked to cancer in lab animals.

• In lab tests on a sunscreen that contained parabens, fish and frogs began to change sex, from male to female.

The Cancer Prevention Coalition, a nonprofit advocacy group, has said, "The cosmetic industry has been as reckless as the tobacco industry and the FDA has remained silent."

Parabens are classified as xenoestrogens, a group of synthetic chemicals that mimic estrogen. Xenoestrogens have been used commercially, on a widespread basis, for decades. In addition to being linked to cancer, they are widely believed to be one of the most prevalent causes of growing infertility rates. Every time you smooth on a paraben-preserved product, you are potentially introducing this chemical into your bloodstream.

But don't worry: That doesn't mean you have to have wrinkly, dry skin, or face the world as bare as the day you were born. There are a growing number of paraben-free products on the market.

Green Guru

Susan Kurz
CEO, DR. HAUSCHKA
MOTHER OF THREE

The very best of the super naturals are by Dr. Hauschka, a line that is not only organic but a step beyond, called biodynamic—that is, produced by a system of agriculture developed by Rudolf Steiner, in which farmers work with the basic principles of nature to bring about balance and healing. Martha Stewart and Brad Pitt are fans of Hauschka's luminous effects. And I can tell you for sure, within six months of my using it, all my friends swore I "had some work done"!

"Hauschka uses all biodynamic, organic extracts in it. Many people have said, 'Oh, I'm allergic to fragrances,' but it's synthetic fragrance that they're normally allergic to. They find they have no problem with our rose or lavender products, because not only are they made from natural ingredients, but because of the agricultural method, there's no synthetic chemicals anywhere along the way.

"But biodynamic means more than synthetic chemical free. Biodynamic also means balance, harmony, and rhythm.

"What's missing from our lives is a sense of rhythm. Everything about our bodies is naturally rhythmical. Your skin renews itself every twenty-eight to forty-two days. There's a rhythm between your blood, your breath, and your heartbeat. We are beings of rhythm, so when we consciously establish rhythms in our lives, it's very empowering, very healing. You can make a ritual out of the things that you have to do anyway. For example, you have to cleanse your skin. So cleanse your skin in the morning, not while thinking about what you have to do in the office, but by being conscious of the fact that you're cleansing your skin, and bringing a rhythmic, compassionate, rolling, pressing motion to the process. You can enhance it by putting a little lavender in the water, which is very good for your whole nervous system. So as you begin your day, the message you give yourself is one of compassion, rhythm, and nurturing. And then that reverberates inward as well as being physically good for your skin.

"Performing rhythmic rituals gives you more time, not less, because it helps you integrate all those different elements in your life that you're trying to keep up with. When you do something that is nurturing, it lifts you up. Then everything else starts to fall into place. If you keep going back to that, you'll find yourself more grounded."

Green Flag

The following paraben-free brands are all available online or at Whole Foods Market and health-food stores:

Dr. Hauschka: www.drhauschka.com
MyChelle: www.mychelleusa.com
Weleda: www.usa.weleda.com
Burt's Bees: www.burtsbees.com
Pangea: www.pangeaorganics.com
Kimberly Sayer: www.kimberlysayer.com
Zia Natural Skincare: www.zianatural.com
John Masters Organics: www.johnmasters.com

Red Flag

methylparaben
propylparaben
ethylparaben
butylparaben

Even at health-food stores, always check for parabens in the ingredients. *READ THE LABELS.*

Unlike with food or drugs, there are few "truth in labeling" laws regarding cosmetics and body-care products. A product can be labeled "all-natural" or "organic" and not be either. Worse yet, companies can disguise harmful ingredients by using the term "proprietary formula" on their label. Phrases like "our secret blend of botanical ingredients" can conceal parabens. If you're unsure, call the company and ask.

PUT ON A HAPPY FACE

You're already beautiful, because you are bringing a new person into the world, a unique and special soul, through your body. Everything about you is in a state of creation—a combination of wonderful and luminous, or fatigued and drained. And skinwise, you may be experiencing tumultuous changes, too, vacillating between baby-bottom perfection and blotchy and broken out. For most of us, our skin is a big part of how we "face the day," so you may be using foundation or cover-up, at least occasionally, during your pregnancy. You'll want to choose wisely to be sure what makes you look good is also good for baby.

Foundations vary wildly, in terms of both price and consistency. Each brand is different, but here's a general rule of thumb: the more liquid a foundation, the greater its absorbency (your skin will "drink" more of it in) and the more parabens it probably contains (parabens act as preservatives, which liquids need, since they naturally break down much faster than oils or powders).

But parabens aren't your only concerns when considering makeup. Colors listed on the labels as "FD&C" and "D&C" are also known as coal-tar colors. Made from bituminous coal, these synthetic tints are common ingredients in most cosmetics with color, and they are listed (depending on the color) by the EPA as "possible human carcinogen" and "probable human carcinogen."

Mineral makeups are clean and popular with natural devotees, but are probably not the best choice when you're expecting. Minerals are metals, and metals are something you'll want to avoid when you're pregnant, since the jury is still out on what might affect babies in utero.

For a finish that's as green as it is flawless, consider Zia or Hauschka. Burt's Bees concealer is also terrific.

THE EYES HAVE IT

Almost every mascara I've looked into includes parabens (and I have the puny transparent eyelashes of a white rabbit, so going mascara free is not an option). I have searched high and low, and here is what I came up with: My fave (as you probably already know) is Hauschka, which miraculously makes my diminutive lashes long, black, and silky (well, not long, but much better than the little stubs nature begrudgingly bestowed on me). If you find Hauschka too pricey, try Lavera Volume Mascara, made with extracts of organic jojoba and wild-rose oils. It's paraben free and heavy metal free and rinses off with any mild cleanser. Lavera also makes the very nicest pencil eyeliners in simple subtle shades, as does natural-cosmetics leader Zia.

SEALED WITH A KISS

It's a good idea to check through all your cosmetics for suspect ingredients when you're expecting, since, as you now know, if you're putting it on, you're putting it in. But you may want to be especially vigilant about lipsticks, since you're likely eating a lot of those. Most glosses are made with lots of petroleum derivatives, so you are, in a very real sense, licking a sort of gasoline. The FD&C colors that give glosses their tints and lipsticks their color can travel in through your mouth, and some cross the placenta. So whether you favor a matte red or a shimmering gloss, if it's a conventional brand, better not pay it any lip service. Consider instead a clean and green brand like PeaceKeeper. Their Lip Paint collection includes nine shades of lipstick and gloss, plus all after-tax profits go to support women's-health initiatives.

There are so many ways to safely pamper yourself when you're pregnant, and the loving, soothing things you do for your skin and your body now can begin to condition you into being a loving and effective mother soon. What's the most basic all-natural beauty product? Olive oil. Yes, that's right: The kind you have in the kitchen is perfect for the bath. Just put some in a spray bottle and use it in the shower or bath and as a lotion after. (Later on, it's OK for your baby, as well.)

Hey, Good-lookin', Whatcha Got Cookin'?

My thanks to Nancy Klein, superhero mother of three and Domestic Diva, who cooked up some marvelous all-natural spa recipes you can use to treat yourself, naturally, at home—plus they won't put any strain on your changing budget.

Organic Spinach and Kale Body Mask
Harvard University researchers say ingesting the potent antioxidant lutein, found in dark green leafy vegetables, may protect the skin from sun damage. There is conjecture that it is also beneficial to apply lutein directly to the surface of the skin. In this recipe the cream gives the added benefit of exfoliating lactic acid.

½ cup washed organic spinach
½ cup washed organic kale (middle stem removed)
¼ cup extra-virgin olive oil
¼ cup organic cream

Puree all ingredients in food processor until smooth. Apply in shower. Rinse with water and gently towel dry.

Frozen Margarita Body Scrub

½ lemon (seeds removed)
2 cups organic cane sugar
¼ cup papaya nectar
juice from 1 grapefruit

Combine the ½ lemon and sugar in food processor and pulse until lemon and sugar are well incorporated. Add other ingredients. Puree together in food processor. Freeze in ice-cube trays. Pop from trays and store in plastic storage bag in freezer. Use in shower as invigorating natural hand-held body scrub. On stressful days body-scrub cubes can be put into the blender for spontaneous virgin-margarita parties. (When you're not pregnant or breast-feeding, add white tequila and Cointreau for emergencies!)

Ginger/Wasabi Foot Wake-up Bath and Ginger Massage Oil

Tingly and spicy, this invigorating footbath will revitalize tired feet and calves and bring soothing relief.

6-inch knob of ginger, grated
1 cup boiling water
1 teaspoon wasabi mustard (available in grocery sushi case or in Asian markets)

Place grated ginger in the boiling water. Seep for 10 minutes. Strain ginger water into a container large enough for both feet. Add wasabi and then fill container with very warm water. Place your feet inside and relax. After soaking, seal in the moisture by massaging feet with ginger massage oil (see below). Make sure to wash hands afterward to avoid spreading wasabi to eyes.

Ginger Massage Oil
2-inch knob of ginger, coarsely chopped
½ cup almond, grape-seed, or olive oil

Blend at high speed until liquefied. Strain into nonbreakable container.

All these beauty products should be refrigerated immediately after preparation and should be used as soon as possible to retain optimum freshness and avoid spoilage.

YOU ARE HOW YOU LOOK?

I didn't get pimply with my first pregnancy—my skin was gorgeous—but I did get really big. I didn't consider myself fat. I was pregnant, after all, and I didn't want my baby to go hungry. When I was hungry, I ate, so she wouldn't have to live off my fat and the toxins it stored. As I gained weight, I got lots of comments on my appearance, even some from total strangers! And one day, when I was six months pregnant, I saw an acquaintance while I was walking the dogs. He waved at me and called across the park, "Boy, you got really fat!" I smiled and said, "No, I'm pregnant!" And he said, "Yeah, but you got fat everywhere!"

My feelings weren't hurt, but I was amazed that for so many

people, the world is one big beauty pageant. Except it's one that we enter without our consent!

What's important is not what anyone else thinks, but how you feel. And I felt really beautiful when I was pregnant. I took advantage of the changes pregnancy brings. The truth is, many women do glow when pregnant, due to natural weight gain and water retention, coupled with improved circulation as your blood vessels and veins relax to accommodate the extra blood (about fifty percent!) flowing through your body. This means pregnancy is an opportunity to play up the radiant star that you are. It was the first time I used smoky pencils around my eyes and also the first time I didn't need under-eye cover-up or blush. All those added hormones plumped up my skin and hollow cheeks, so I looked far younger and fresher than my years.

When you're expecting, it's important to embrace your changing beauty, whatever that means to you. Meet one gorgeous woman, below, who will share her tips to help you do just that.

Green Guru

Karim Orange
CELEBRITY MAKEUP ARTIST
MOM

Orange Loves Green
Celebrity makeup artist Karim Orange has worked with superstars, including Aretha Franklin and the Dixie Chicks, and has been nominated for two Emmy Awards for her makeup work

on the smart vixens of *The View*. She's a glossy-magazine favorite because of her unique blending of a down-to-earth, natural approach with va-va-voom glamour.

"Pregnancy can be one of the most beautiful times for most women, not just on a physical level, but spiritually and emotionally, as well. We all know to eat plenty of organic fruits and vegetables. Avocados are a terrific source of heart-healthy fat and do wonders for the skin before, during, and after pregnancy. Avocados also have the highest amount of dietary fiber, by weight, of any fruit. (That's right, they're fruits!) Avocados are one of the best sources of glutathione, a major antioxidant that has been shown to retard a number of cancers; they're also a good source of vitamin C.

"If you're having skin issues when you're expecting, please remember that during this time your body is responding to a lot of hormonal changes. Continue taking (under doctor supervision) your essential fatty acids (EFAs). I love The Essential Woman by Barlean's, which has the proper blends of omega-3-6-9 plus primrose. All these ingredients make skin glow from the inside out.

"Try the following for specific skin-care issues; everything recommended is organic and free of parabens. I love the brand Pangea, whose products are so exotic. It's great to indulge when you're pregnant!

• Puffy eyes: Drink more water and eat less salt. Place cucumber slices on your eyes in the morning, or try cold chamomile tea bags, which will have a calming effect. Also try Evan Healy's Chamomile Eye Care Cream.

• Breakouts: Your EFAs will help with this. Also try Pangea Organics' Japanese Matcha Tea with Acai & Goji Berry Facial Mask.

• Dry skin: Try Pangea Organics' Italian Red Mandarin with Roses Facial Cream.

• Total skin freak-out (dry today, oily tomorrow): Try Pangea Nigerian Ginger, Sweet Lavender & Thyme Facial Cream.

"If you want to use makeup while pregnant, please make sure it is all-natural, such as Dr. Hauschka, Zuzu Luxe, or Gabriel. Stick with nonmineral makeup during pregnancy. I like products that are vegan, organic, or both.

"Every ethnic group has its issues and concerns. African-Americans tend not to get wrinkles until late in life—you know the old saying 'Black don't crack'—but we do tend to have oily skin and hyperpigmentation and we don't use as much sunscreen as we should. But everyone's skin responds to the same things: proper diet, low stress, and common-sense earth-, animal-, and people-friendly products."

GREEN AT A GLANCE

Evergreen: Dump all your conventional beauty products. Go totally green with a super program from brands like Dr. Hauschka, Weleda, or MyChelle.

Pea green: Make your own skin and beauty treatments. This is very cost-effective, and you know there won't be any parabens in those!

Spring green: Swap out the things you use most often, like facial moisturizer and hand lotion, for clean and natural brands.

Three

Head, Shoulders, Nails, and Toes!

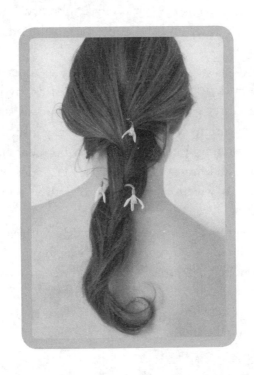

From Hair Salons and Hair Dye to the Truth About Mani-pedis

I can almost guarantee that your hair will change when you're pregnant. Many women experience the most luscious locks of their lives when they're expecting, while others are losing chunks by the fistful. If you're in the first group, congratulations! If you're in the second, don't worry—it's only temporary, and with the delivery of your beautiful baby, your bountiful head of hair will begin to return.

In my case (lucky me!) my mane became as super sumptuous as Lady Godiva's. My hair thickened as fast as my bottom, so much so that catty girlfriends gossiped that I was splurging on weaves and extensions (not true). But you may just as easily find your tresses thinning. Either way, it's your hormones to thank or to rail against, and most of the changes you notice in your hair during pregnancy will abate within six to twelve weeks after your baby arrives.

In the meantime, how can you best deal with your feast or famine? Of course a good cut is the best way to start. Now might be a good time to go shorter. A lower-maintenance cut can look fresh and chic and could do a lot for someone else's self-confidence, too! How? See below for a glimpse of how your shorn tresses can continue turning heads.

TAKE IT OFF—TAKE IT ALL OFF Kathy Semke, a hair-stylist in Irvington, New York, is a twenty-five-year veteran of the beauty trade, and one of the most sought-after stylists in swanky Westchester County. Semke says many of her expectant clients choose to go shorter and blunt, in part because a good blunt cut will make even corn-silk-thin hair seem thick and swingy. Another reason for them to take it off: Semke works in conjunction with Locks of Love, a nonprofit organization that will turn shorn tresses into wigs for children who have lost their hair, sometimes from going through chemotherapy treatments for cancer. "It can be a relief to get rid of long hair, but it can be a little sad, too," says Semke. "After all, that hair has been with you a long time! With Locks of Love, clients just feel so happy and free. They understand that their loss really is someone else's gain!"

To see how fab other donors' tresses look on recipients, check out the moving and inspirational pictures on www.locksoflove.org.

But what about color? You've probably heard you shouldn't color your hair when you're pregnant, because the chemicals can be bad for your growing baby. Ugh! With all the other lifestyle changes you're making, do you have to abandon that, too? Now when you're feeling all dumpy and fat? There are alternatives that can keep your baby safe, and keep you from looking like Cruella De Vil.

The Environmental Working Group, a nonprofit consumer-advocacy group, recently found that no less than seventy-one percent of all commercial hair-dye products, most of which are available in the United States, contain ingredients derived from carcinogenic coal tar. It also found that out of more than ten thousand chemicals used in personal-care products, only about eleven percent have been assessed by the government for safety.

It's important that you avoid strong-smelling chemical treatments, like perms and Japanese straightening. Full-head color is also not recommended, especially permanent color (semipermanent has fewer chemicals) and dark colors (which are more likely to have higher tar concentrations).

Red Flag
perms
permanent full-head color (at the salon or at home)
any ammonia-based treatment or color

Green Guru

John Masters
FOUNDER, JOHN MASTERS SALON

In a beautiful storefront salon on a historic street in Manhattan's posh SoHo district, there's a revolution going on—an environmental revolution—and it's called John Masters Organics. When you open the salon's door, you're met by a heavy velvet curtain. Pull that back and walk into a world of peace and beauty. John is a pioneer in the natural-products movement, having been involved in cleaner beauty for seventeen years.

"I think caring about yourself and caring about the earth don't have to be mutually exclusive. I spent years honing my skills at a classic, chic salon on Fifth Avenue. But I started living my life more holistically, and as I was changing everything else, I began to wonder why I was breathing in all these toxic fumes. I asked myself, 'What am I doing?' and left. I wanted to make a haven where getting beautiful was not a grueling or unhealthy experience.

"But I could only cut so much hair every day, and only so many people have access to appointments at the salon, so I went a step further, and began to formulate my beauty 'concoctions' into a line. First hair care, then a full beauty-care line, John Masters Organics.

"We only get one body, and we only get one planet. Why not treat them both with the utmost care? I didn't want to deal with chemicals and synthetics every day, and I truly believed that when given the option, others would feel the same. Why use synthetics when natural products work better and are safer for the environment?

"I get lots of soon-to-be moms in here. We're a clean-air salon, which means no permanents, no chemical hair straightening. As far as hair coloring goes, we use the safest, ammonia-free, herbal-based dyes, with the lowest amount of PPDs (a carcinogen). Still, for expectant women, full-head hair color is probably not the way to go. Instead, you could choose highlights or lowlights. The key is for the product not to touch the scalp, because you don't want the dye to be absorbed by your skin.

"We use a terrific new product from L'Oréal called Illumin, which has no PPDs, ammonia, or peroxide. If your colorist is skillful enough, you shouldn't have to have highlights more than two or three times during your whole pregnancy.

"At the moment, we don't sell any color treatments outside the salon, so I'm going to give you my recipe for the most natural highlights that you can make and use at home."

John Masters' Make-It-at-Home Natural Highlights

Brew 2 bags of chamomile tea in 2 cups water; strain and let cool. Squeeze in fresh lemon juice. (Use the juice of at least 2 lemons, more if you have a lot of hair.) Pour the mixture over clean hair. Do not rinse. Sunlight will accelerate the lightening process, so for the fastest results, put this mixture in a spray bottle and pack it in your bag when you head to the shore! The more often you spritz, the more highlights you'll see.

THE PLUSES AND MINUSES OF IONS; *OR, HOW YOUR HAIRDRYER MAY AFFECT YOUR MOOD*

OK, at the risk of sounding really hippie-dippie, here goes. Your hair dryer may be bumming you out, man. (And likewise your computer terminal, and for that matter your air conditioner.) And it's not just me and Cheech and Chong asserting this—these vibes we're picking up are supported by scientific data, too.

A negative ion is, generally speaking, a molecule with an extra electron.

Molecules with extra electrons elicit feelings of well-being in people exposed to them. They are found in large quantities on ocean beaches, and such. "The action of the pounding surf creates negative air ions, and we also see it immediately after spring thunderstorms, when people report lightened moods," says ion researcher Michael Terman, PhD, of Columbia University in New York.

Although negative ions are plentiful in nature (think forests and waterfalls), they are usually lacking in the workplace, especially in hair salons using conventional dryers.

Positive ions are also found in nature, and have long been known to produce feelings of anxiety. In Native American mythology, California's seasonal Santa Ana winds were known as "the bitter winds" and were thought to bring with them depression and sleepless nights. In the south of France, similarly, the mistral winds are said to usher in unhappiness and chaos. (Winston Churchill avoided visiting the Mediterranean coast when the mistral was blowing.) All these winds are very dry, with very low humidity. So you may be doing your own version of a wrathful Mother Nature with your hair dryer if it's conventional; you're positioning a very hot dry wind—charged with positive ions—at your head every day. Need a Prozac with that new do?

Help is at hand, however. There are ionic hair dryers that emit millions of negative ions via ceramic plates. In addition to producing negative ions, ceramic ionic dryers dry hair up to sixty percent faster and help it hold in moisture. (That's making me feel better already!)

Salons—and expecting moms—should also look for hair dryers that reduce electromagnetic fields (EMFs). Excessive exposure to EMFs was linked in a 1998 U.S. government report to increased levels of leukemia in children and adults.

Green Flag

There are great natural products from shampoo to tints for "clean," green hair (no, not the color green):

Max Green Alchemy: some of the finest and cleanest shampoos and hair-care products on the market, with no synthetic additives or petrochemicals

Surya Nature: completely natural hennas and hair color
Tints of Nature: ammonia-free permanent and semipermanent at-home hair color
Aubrey Organics: reasonably priced and very clean

THE LONG AND SHORT OF IT—NAIL SALONS

True, you might not be able to see your toes, but it sure would feel good to have a soak and a foot rub. How hot can the water be? And what about the formaldehyde in the nail polish and toxins in the remover? Do you have to give up every luxury? Or can you just plow forward and forget a few little indiscretions? Come with me on a trip to a magical land, where puffy pregnant feet are pampered and no corners are cut on baby's well-being.

Green Guru

Kim D'Amato
FOUNDER AND OWNER, PRITI ORGANIC SPA
MOM

On a little treelined side street deep in Manhattan's East Village, taxis pull up by the dozens every day to deposit some of the city's most beautiful and in-the-know folks at the tiny, feng-shuied storefront that houses Priti Organic Spa. In a city that boasts hundreds, maybe thousands, of chic places that cater to the well-coiffed woman's right to buff and polish, what's so special about Priti? Well, just about everything.

"Eight years ago when I was expecting my daughter, I found myself interested in organics and began taking notice of what I was doing to myself, my body, and my soon-to-be-born baby. While visiting a nail salon and breathing the less-than-fresh air, I wondered how exposure to these chemicals might be harming me, my child, and other expectant mothers. I kept thinking, there must be a way to have your nails done without exposing yourself to chemicals. So I set about trying to build a spa that wouldn't expose you to all those toxins. If I can buy organic foods, I should be able to buy organic beauty products.

"In my research, I learned just how dangerous some of those chemicals are.

"Dibutyl phthalate—otherwise known as DBP—is a plasticizer used in nail polish to create that smooth, polished finish we all love. In a study, the Centers for Disease Control raised a red flag when every woman in the study had DBP present in her body; the highest levels showed up in women of childbearing age. According to the CDC, 'DBP is known to harm the male reproductive system. It causes birth defects of testicular atrophy, reduced sperm count, and defects in the structure of the penis.'

"Formaldehyde, a carcinogen linked to cancer of the nose and throat, and toluene, a chemical known to harm unborn babies, are standard ingredients in most nail polishes.

"And, of course, parabens, which have been linked to cancer, are found in most face creams and beauty products.

"At Priti, we use organic body and beauty products, including organic sugar scrubs to safely slough off dry skin, and clean nail polishes that have no formaldehyde, DBP, or toluene. In our facial room we use Dr. Alkaitis Holistic Organic Skin Food. We use soy nail-polish remover.

"I honestly believe that organic products do not have to cost too much. People are scared of organics because they associate them with the word 'expensive.' But it's quite simple and inexpensive to do organic treatments at home.

"Organic sugar scrubs are made using organic sugar, organic essential oils, and carrier oils. They are very inexpensive and easy to make. Add a couple of drops of each oil to a quarter cup of sugar, and that's it. Or soak in a bath of warm water and your favorite organic essential oil, plus a few rose petals!

"With nontoxic nail polish, you can do your mani and pedi in the comfort of your own home. So put your feet up and spend some time in luxury."

If you still want to visit a regular manicurist, follow these simple guidelines:

- Skip the polish and consider a good filing and buffing.

- Use formaldehyde-free nail polish. (You might need to take your own.)

- Choose one or the other—hands or feet—and ask if you can sit in the best-ventilated seat.

- Limit your time—and your skin's exposure—in the chemical air of the nail salon. Call ahead to check when they're least busy. Schedule an appointment then: You won't have to wait, and there will be fewer chemicals in the air when there are fewer clients.

Neat Feet and Happy Hands

Here are some tips from green-beauty-industry pioneer Firozé, renowned for her expertise in mani-pedis. She also has her own formaldehyde-free nail-polish line (of the same name).

Soothing Treatment for Rough Heels

Combine 2 tablespoons honey, 1 teaspoon baking soda, and 1 tablespoon almond oil. Mix well. Apply generously to the soles of feet, then slide feet into heavy socks. Sleep with mixture on and wash it off in the morning.

If you are unable to sleep with mask overnight, leave it on for a minimum of 30 minutes, then wash it off. For people who have especially cracked heels, this treatment should be repeated 2 to 3 times a week for the ideal results.

To Pamper Nails, Cuticles, and Skin on Your Hands and Feet

Heat 1 cup olive oil in a pan until it is just warm. Squeeze the juice of 1 fresh lemon into the warm olive oil and . . . you have yourself a salad dressing! Yes, it is natural and good enough to eat, but this treat is for your nails and hands.

Soak in this delicious warm mixture for 20 minutes to soften your skin, fade sunspots and liver spots, and whiten and strengthen your nails. Most importantly, it will take care of your nails' best friend: your cuticles.

GREEN AT A GLANCE

Evergreen: Use John's chamomile spray in lieu of traditional highlights.

Pea green: Give up the standard mani-pedi and give yourself a home treatment.

Spring green: Choose only highlights and book an appointment during a not-too-busy time.

Four

Makes
Scents

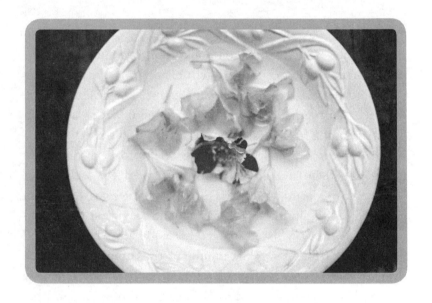

Perfumes and Synthetic Fragrances

Fragrances are a multibillion-dollar industry, but research indicates that we may need to rethink what we are putting on our bodies, especially when we are pregnant. There is substantial evidence that synthetic fragrances are related to a variety of conditions, ranging from headaches and nausea to birth defects.

I really went "off the scent" walking along Broadway one warm spring day when I was five months pregnant. I was walking (or waddling) up toward Macy's at Thirty-fourth Street to have them put another link in my Movado watchband. My wrist was straining against my watchband like a Thoroughbred when you pull back on the reins. It was the middle of the morning, and back then, that was not a residential neighborhood, so it was mostly me and bike messengers and folks in cars. All of a sudden I became very, very nauseous. A sickeningly sweet scent descended upon me and clung to the spring breeze. Ahhh! I saw the perpetrator. She was across the street and up two blocks. I had to turn back. If I couldn't stand that woman's cologne on the street, from blocks away, I knew I'd never make it through the main floor of Macy's.

Your nose knows. If you can smell it, it is entering your bloodstream. And chances are, it is not too natural.

So before you plunk down the plastic on the glass countertop at Saks or Bloomie's, you may want to consider the following.

NATURAL SELECTION

It makes sense to avoid synthetic scents. Ninety-five percent of all perfume or fragrance ingredients are derived from petroleum and contain phthalates. Phthalates are a group of chemicals used to soften plastics and bind chemicals. They are present in every synthetic fragrance and are linked to a variety of serious health disorders, including severe allergies, asthma, and even cancer. Phthalates give off volatile organic compounds, known as VOCs, which are also found in vapors emitted from products like toxic solvents, wood preservatives, paint strippers, and dry-cleaning chemicals.

VOCs are known to produce eye, nose, and throat irritation, as well as headaches, loss of coordination, nausea, liver damage, and harm to the kidneys and the central nervous system, according to the Environmental Protection Agency. Some VOCs can cause cancer in animals and are suspected or known to cause cancer in humans.

In olden times, perfume was so wonderful and so expensive because it really came only from flower petals, lots and lots of flower petals. Now most fragrances are made in the lab, and unbelievable as it may sound, most ingredients are never tested for safety.

These toxic substances can be especially harmful because they enter the bloodstream two different ways: you put them on your skin, and you also breathe them in.

Red Flag

Hundreds of studies on animals have shown that phthalates can damage the liver, kidneys, lungs, and reproductive system, especially the developing testes.

Phthalates are found in many leading beauty-care products, including the hair spray, deodorant, nail polish, and fragrance that you may be using every day.

A 2000 study on children's health in the medical journal *Environmental Health Perspectives* found a link between premature breast development in young girls (under the age of nine) and phthalates in the bloodstream. "This is a serious public health anomaly," the journal reported. "The phthalates we have identified have been classified as endocrine disruptors. This study suggests a possible association between plasticizers with known estrogenic and antiandrogenic activity and premature breast development in the human female."

A November 2002 study by the Harvard University School of Public Health found a link between sperm damage and monoethyl phthalate, a compound used to maintain the color and scent in many cosmetic items such as perfumes, colognes, and hair spray.

The European Union has banned two types of phthalates. The U.S. government has failed to take similar action. Until it does, you should avoid synthetic fragrances as much as possible, and ask those around you (and those who will be around your baby) to do the same.

Keep in mind that you won't find phthalates listed on the labels, because the chemical formulas of fragrances are considered "trade secrets" and makers are not required to disclose them. Check out the Environmental Working Group's site www.nottoopretty.com for a comprehensive listing of popular cosmetics and fragrances, and a grading system on their toxicity levels.

Green Flag
Your nose knows and probably common sense (or common scents) will lead the way. Chances are your "obsession" with a certain

fragrance evaporated with your pregnancy. Some clean and healthy alternatives that keep you smelling like a rose:

- www.kuumbamade.com

- www.sunrosearomatics.com

- www.homespaorganics.com

Green Guru

Kuumba
KUUMBA MADE

I met Kuumba at a press event in Manhattan where the toniest brands were touting their unique properties to some of the most influential fashion editors in the world. Something about her down-to-earth manner and inner confidence radiated warmth and beauty. Her personality was like a magnet . . . or was it that captivating fragrance? Kuumba's healing salve is a must-have for any medicine cabinet. It does double duty as a cure for (ugh!) hemorrhoids and minor itchies, such as bug bites. It's petroleum free and safe for kids, too.

"Kuumba Made started in 1980 when I learned from a friend in the West Indies how to make coconut oil: You crack the coconut, shake it, and squeeze out the oil by hand. It's a beautiful process and makes a beautiful product. Coconut oil is one of the best things you can apply to your skin, and of course it smells wonderful. There is a mystical quality to natural fragrances. The same things that attract birds and bees attract people, too. Scent is one of our most primal and undisturbed senses. The coconut is so soothing, and it keeps you from getting stretch marks. After giving birth, lots of moms stick with it because it's such a superb moisturizer. Sometimes I mix it with other fragrances, such as ground-up rose petals or lavender. Natural fragrances energize. They have a tremendous draw, and the attractive energy of these products is amazing. I apprenticed as an herbalist and grew organic gardens for twenty years. I've found that often what you need is growing right outside your door. The earth gives us everything we need to live beautiful, healthy lives. Herbs and flowers are the real medicines, and will heal us."

BECAUSE YOU'RE WORTH IT

To reduce your exposure to phthalates, you don't have to go totally au naturel. Instead, opt for fragrances that are phthalate free, or have lower amounts in their ingredients. Since the EU ban on two widely used kinds of phthalates, suspected of contributing to birth defects, Revlon and L'Oréal have stepped up and developed some phthalate-free products. Also, you can always count on Aveda for phthalate-free or low-phthalate products, and The Body Shop has some wonderful items that are super-fragrant and phthalate free.

To stay sweet smelling but toxin free, keep this in mind: As a general rule, perfumes usually have far lower doses of phthalates than their cologne cousins. For example, Chanel No. 5 and No. 19 are relatively phthalate free. Essential oils are best because they are just that—oils made from the plant, flower, or herb they smell like—and don't contain any of the chemical burdens of synthetic scents.

And what if you are more "personally fragrant" than usual? Yes, besides the odd sounds that may be escaping your body, you may also be noticing other less-than-appealing symptoms of your impending happy event, thanks to the changes your body is going through and your accompanying increased hormones. Switching from a conventional underarm deodorant or antiperspirant to a natural one is an easy way to reduce your exposure to phthalates. Aerosol sprays are the worst when it comes to phthalates. Use a roll-on or stick instead. Here are the best: the Green Salt Stick, Tom's of Maine, Desert Essence, and my fave, Weleda.

COME ON, BABY, LIGHT MY FIRE

I love a great candle. Maybe it's because I used to be a smoker. In fact, smoking was my first true love. (Make that second. Grape-flavored Now and Later candies were my first, though we had a nasty breakup when they pulled my braces off. . . .) Smoking probably sounds super gross if you're pregnant and have never smoked. Or it sounds super appealing if you used to be a smoker and, like me, quit cold turkey for the sake of your beautiful bump. But either way, you, too, probably feel there is something wonderful and soothing about flame and fragrance. And it's amazing, even a little magical, to see something emit light. A candle is a mini refuge, a welcome luxury, and a nice addition to your life.

Unless it is (cue ominous drumroll) the candle that kills! Or at the very least, the one that makes you cough.

There are several potential dangers in fragranced candles.

The wick. Many expensive fragranced candles have a metal core in their wicks. A metal core keeps a cotton wick from flipping over and extinguishing itself in a pool of wax. But burning metal is never a good thing; some wicks even have a lead core, which is downright dangerous.

The fragrance. If it's synthetic, your "watermelon wave" is a veritable tsunami, carrying phthalates everywhere you can smell it. So all that we talked about in the beginning of the chapter related to scents, you are putting into every breath you take.

The wax. Paraffin is a petroleum-based by-product of refined gasoline. When paraffin is burned, it releases carcinogenic toxins into the air.

Red Flag

Experts from the American Lung Association say that candles are fast becoming one of the most common unrecognized causes of poor indoor-air quality.

According to Jerome O. Nriagu, PhD, a professor of environmental chemistry at the University of Michigan in Ann Arbor, burning as little as four metal-wick candles for two hours can result in airborne lead concentrations that pose a distinct and direct threat to human health.

Green Flag

Unlike for cigarettes, there are safe alternatives for candles, and the natural ones are much more luxurious and enjoyable than their toxic cousins.

• Beeswax candles were the norm before they were replaced by those made from tallow and paraffin. But check the label: A product only has to contain more than fifty percent beeswax to be labeled a beeswax candle (and the rest can be paraffin).

• Soy candles are made from soybean oil, a type of vegetable oil. Safe and smooth-burning.

The best natural candles will be paraffin free and also free of synthetic fragrances. You need to check every candle you buy, because some makers of the aromatic soy candles are still using synthetic fragrances.

Green Guru

John Kornbluh
FOUNDER, BLUECORN NATURALS

If, like me, you loved the episode of *Mr. Rogers' Neighborhood* when he actually showed how and where crayons were made, you'll relish this story about Bluecorn Naturals candles. And how one man's need became a beautiful business.

"In the winter of 1991 in a one-room cabin in Telluride, Colorado, I dipped my first beeswax candle. Necessity is the mother of invention, and the mother of my business. I was a ski bum and living in a cabin with no utilities (and a very frosty outhouse) when I started getting really bad headaches. A friend told me it might be the kerosene lamp I burned every night and that I should switch to candles. He got me a bucket and some beeswax and I started to dip. My headaches disappeared, and I was hooked! In many ways, my business hasn't changed so much since those early days. It's still about simplicity. Every candle we make is still hand dipped here in Colorado. We have 6 employees in a town of 250. I think we're the largest employer in town.

"We make soy and all kinds of natural candles, but beeswax

is the best. The wax is excreted by bees from a gland under their wings. It's what they build their comb from. Everything happens in the comb, the birthing of baby bees, the making of honey; it's their home. A bee will fill a comb with honey and cap it with wax. A beekeeper only takes the wax from the cap: he never destroys the comb. The bees simply remake the cap. A busy bee is a happy bee and a beekeeper has a vested interest in keeping the bees happy. Their lives are good. It's the ultimate in sustainability.

"Beeswax has the highest melting point of any wax, so beeswax candles have the longest burn time. It's a superclean-burning wax. Paraffin, on the other hand, is a petroleum by-product; its emissions are similar to those that come from diesel fuel.

"Never go for paraffin. Remember, you breathe what you burn!"

GREEN AT A GLANCE

Evergreen: Stop using conventional deodorants or anti-perspirants. Switch to a natural alternative: a salt stick, or a product by Weleda or Desert Essence.

Pea green: Stop wearing cologne or heavily fragranced products at least for the duration of your pregnancy, and ask your mate to do the same.

Spring green: Choose natural candles with nonmetal wicks. And choose perfumes with the lowest amount of phthalates.

Five

Green
Baby Shower

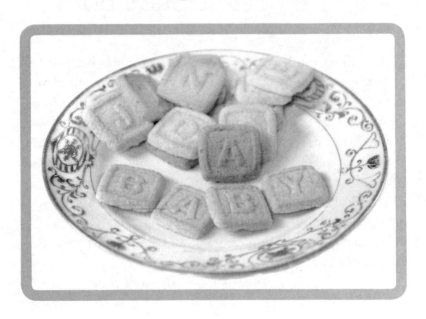

How to Have the Most
Fun with Your Baby,
Even Before She's Born

Hopefully you have a great friend or close relative who will help you out by offering to throw a bash in honor of your expected. My gorgeous and glamorous sister, Dawn Bridges, did for me, and it was dreamy. She knew me so well it was filled with wonderful surprises. (The games below come from her ingenuity.) But if you're separated from your family by distance, and your girlfriends aren't too forthcoming, drop a few hints. If they don't pick up the ball, throw the shower yourself. You and your baby deserve it!

Here's how to make it memorable and ensure you're not wasting lots of Mother Earth's resources.

Let your friends and guests know ahead of time how you'd most like them to help you celebrate the new life you're expecting.

Right now is your opportunity to start living your new lifestyle, your green dream.

E-mailing invites cuts down on many forms of waste, but if you want a classic with a twist, consider recycled paper. Producing recycled white paper creates seventy-four percent fewer air pollutants and thirty-five percent fewer water pollutants, and uses seventy-five percent less process energy, than producing paper from virgin fibers. Or send your invites via postcard, which uses only half as much paper as a card and an envelope.

You might want to tell friends you're interested in natural parenting, and register at some of the following sites:

- www.kidbean.com

- www.babybunz.com

- www.thenaturalnewborn.com

- www.ourgreenhouse.com

- www.itsonlynatural.us

Perhaps you don't want to burden a friend who might be watching the "green." Let her know you'd love to receive hand-made coupons for, say, two hours of babysitting or a home-cooked meal. (Just let her know when you plan on cashing one in, and don't ask her to cook a meal for eight!)

Make sure people know you would welcome items that have been used and loved. A washed and folded wardrobe of tried-and-true duds can be a real godsend when your baby outgrows all those newborn ensembles.

When I was expecting my second child, a thoughtful but un-employed friend brought me a beautiful poem about the life my daughter would have and her wishes for it. It was the best gift, out of many wonderful ones, that I got that day!

This is your day, a chance for you to express yourself and ask for the world the way you really want it to be.

Remember, you are the queen. Magnanimous and magnifi-cent. In the natural world, there is no creature more revered than the expectant female.

THE DECORATIONS

If you're thinking of using flowers either for the place settings or the centerpiece, consider buying organic ones. Your flowers will certainly be admired, handled, sniffed, and displayed, and conventionally grown ones may contain many times the amount of chemicals allowed on food. (I shudder to think about all the times I brought a sick friend an armful of pesticide-laced flowers: Hope you feel better, buddy! Ahhhhchooo!)

For blooms that are truly as beautiful as they look, check out www.organicbouquet.com or www.diamondorganics.com.

THE WRAPPING-PAPER CONUNDRUM

One of the most wasteful things about a baby shower (or any occasion with presents) is the wrapping paper. About four million tons of waste each year is attributed to wrapping paper! So in the couple of seconds it takes to tear through that colorful stuff to get to the goodies, we are creating a toxic legacy that will soon land in the dump. To make matters worse, many of the finishes that give the wrapping paper its gloss and sheen are highly toxic. Glimmering metallics are the most environmentally offensive, containing, not surprisingly, metal compounds and sometimes even lead.

If you like, ask for unwrapped gifts, or subtly suggest that gifts could be combined and wrapped in another gift, like a crib blanket, cloth diapers, or burp pads. If only paper wrapping will do, there's the old standby of the Sunday funnies, or consider a more unconventional approach: Suggest to guests that they might check out what books your local library is sending to the landfill. Up to forty percent of the used books donated to libraries end up in the Dumpster; their pages might be damaged, or their contents outdated. Choose colorful coffee table photo books, or glossy book covers, and tape them together to make conversation-inspiring and highly original gift wrap—it's super-economical, too! (My daughter used to find old maps especially appealing. She loved looking for the names of former Soviet-bloc countries.)

ALL TIED UP

I like to tie gifts with jute from the hardware store. Jute is natural and sustainable and also surprisingly beautiful. Plus, if you save it, a good piece will come in handy in so many different ways.

Another colorful way to spruce up a gift: tassels and ribbons made out of T-shirts you no longer wear.

To make a T-shirt tassel, cut three-inch fringe along the bottom of a bright shirt, then cut it all off two inches above the highest point of the fringe. (This will make four or five tassels.) Cut your fringe trim into strips that are about five inches wide. Cut a one-inch-wide strip off what is now the bottom of the shirt to gather the fringe and make your tassel. Cut more one-inch-wide strips until you have enough to use as your "ribbon" to tie the package together. This is an easy, no-sew project that anyone can do. You can make a bunch at a time to keep on hand. The tassels look terrific on a bottle of wine, too. (When you're giving a gift to a not-pregnant friend!)

OK, let the shower games begin!

TASTING IS BELIEVING!

A great green baby-shower game is to blindfold your guests and offer them spoonfuls of three different conventional jarred baby foods. Participants then guess the flavors, which proves surprisingly difficult. Next, ask them to try three organic baby foods. The tastes are so distinctive that some of your friends may become green converts!

WHAT'S IN A NAME?

Give each guest a piece of paper and a pencil and a healthy handful or two of Earth's Best organic Letter of the Day cookies. Set the kitchen timer for five minutes and see how many names (real or totally made-up) each guest can spell out of the letters on the cookies. (The vanilla flavor is so amazing, like a shortbread cookie, you may find guests coming up with a full mouth and only short names like Al or Mo.)

INSTANT RECYCLING: THE MUMMY TUMMY GAME

After opening your presents, take the leftover ribbons and tie them together to make one long string. Next, pass the ribbon among the guests, and ask them to guess how much length it will take to go around the honoree's expanded tummy. Use a pen to mark each guest's guess and her initials on the ribbon. When everyone has guessed, gently encircle Mom-to-be with the ribbon and see who wins! The winner receives a little gift, and Mom gets to keep the mummy tummy ribbon as a reminder of when she was so very grand!

THE EATS

The best choices for power-packed snacking will please the most discerning palates; the boost of antioxidants they provide will keep baby going strong, too. A salad made from in-season organic fruits is perfect. The hostess doesn't need to go crazy on the rest; light nosh foods are fun for afternoon parties. The yummiest (and most convenient) munchies are from Newman's Own, Garden of Eatin', or Walnut Acres. Farmer Steve's organic all-natural microwave popcorn is always a huge hit, and a healthy twist on a snack-food classic.

Green Guru

Courtney Fuchs
OWNER, IT'S ONLY NATURAL
(ECOBOUTIQUE AND GIFT STORE)

Sometimes you know someone who just knows how to do everything so it looks at once fresh yet comforting. Someone who's forward thinking, but not "way out there" or inappropriate. Sound like the perfect person to throw your baby shower? Meet Courtney.

"A baby shower is a new beginning for both the parents and the baby. It presents a great opportunity for the party planner and party guests to expand their minds and reconsider how they normally do things. From the invitations to the gifts and decor, everything can be done a little more environmentally, with attention to how your celebration affects the planet.

"Start with the invitations. Consider using cards that are made either from paper with recycled content or from more unusual tree-free—and beautiful—sources, such as hemp, kenaf, or denim scraps. One of my favorites is hand-pressed *lokta* paper. Any of these papers will add a beautiful feel to your invitation instead of a processed, mass-produced feel.

"Keep the decor true to your eco-minded mode. Consider options that are not throwaway or onetime-use items. Small pots of green or flowering plants (organic of course!) can be set around the room or grouped on the food table, then given to the guests as party favors. Place the plants in small baskets, or if you want to have some creative fun, buy plain terra-cotta pots and paint them with the baby-shower date and a design to match the theme, such as baby footprints, flowers, or bees. (Use sponge stamps if you aren't da Vinci.)

"Your centerpiece can be the pièce de résistance! Consider using a widemouthed ceramic vase with a tall base, or a fair trade basket. Fill it with organic, nontoxic baby things: rolled-up diapers, wooden rattles, classic books, burp cloths, and baby-friendly bath goods. Have fun creating a festive arrangement! The pot or basket can be used later as a nice—and useful—reminder of the day."

THE GIFT THAT KEEPS ON GIVING (AND BEING REUSED)

At the end of your shindig, give all the guests a nice bag of goodies that reflect your green taste. Sharon Rowe of Eco-Bags (www.eco bags.com) says, "I love giving reusable bags as gifts. My favorite for gifting is my organic-cotton fold-over bag. It's actually made to be a kids' reusable lunch bag, but it's the perfect size for a goody bag. It's only seven dollars, and it can later be put to work carrying organic meals when you're on the go. If I have the time and am feeling really creative, I use a nontoxic permanent marker to inscribe something memorable on the bag. That way my friend can remember the occasion and my good feelings whenever she uses it."

IN THE BAG

Make sure to give your best buddies extra-special treats. (Remember, you're going to want a trusted babysitter every now and then!)

Priya Haji of World of Good (www.worldofgood.com) has some terrific ideas for small but meaningful gifts to help guests remember this special occasion: "I love our collection of hand-made gift boxes created by women using innovative materials: recycled candy wrappers, small mirrors, and even leaf litter! The great thing about fair trade is that most of the artisans are women—mothers just like us—who invest the increased earn-ings in their children's future. Another one of my favorites is our 'opening doors' key ring, which is made by artisans in Kenya. The proceeds help unlock a brighter future for children through educational scholarships. What better gift at a baby shower than one that opens new possibilities in the life of a child living half a world away?"

A GOOD WORD There's no need to panic, because it's all going to be wonderful—but you will have your hands full when baby arrives. So now, while you have the time, and the free hands, why not write your thank-yous and slip them in the goody bags? After all, what you're really grateful for is not the gifts your friends and loved ones brought to the shower, but the gifts they bring every day by being in your life. (My favorites are the beautiful "note of thanks" collection from TheRoosterCrows.com, where your purchase helps ensure medi-cal care for the family's daughter Anne, who suffers from environmen-tal disease.)

If you can't think of the right words to express how you feel, a general but sincere "I love you and am so happy you'll be in my child's life" will mean a lot. Your friends will forgive you for being mushy as they wipe a tear from their eyes; after all, you've got those raging mommy hormones.

GREEN AT A GLANCE

Evergreen: Register at a green site, such as www.kidbean.com or www.itsonlynatural.us, to ensure all baby's gifts will be best for Mother Earth.

Pea green: Ask guests to please forgo the paper wrapping and use items like a baby blanket or cloth diapers as wrapping.

Spring green: If you choose to register at a conventional store, consider doubling up. If you get two of something, donate one to a local homeless shelter. Forty percent of the inhabitants at shelters are children. You won't be cutting down on waste, but you'll feel good about helping a baby who is not as lucky as yours.

Six 🍃

Mean Green Cleaning Machine

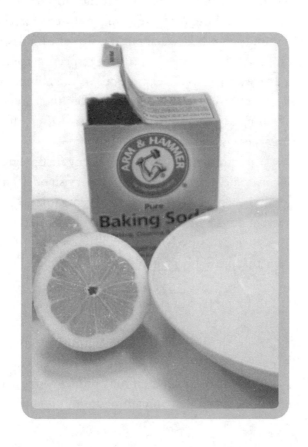

The Safe Way to
Get Ready for Baby

I've always enjoyed a rather "relaxed" attitude toward household cleaning. Ask my husband: He'll solemnly concur that the dust bunnies under our bed are about the size of tumbleweeds. I often took to heart the Japanese custom of respecting spiders and the webs they weave as artistic expressions of the mystery of life. (Now, really, how could I sweep that away from the corner of the ceiling?) Cleaning the bathtub? Maybe later—after all, where there is water, there is life!

However, deep into the third trimester of my first pregnancy, a change came over me. I became a whirling dervish of clean. I was driven to scrub, sweep, vacuum, dust, even reorganize. I had succumbed to the famous nesting instinct. I was enamored with Mr. Clean. And no wonder—we had so much in common! We both wanted to get that little bit of gook out from the corner of the kitchen floor.

And you can be pretty sure that if it happened to me, it will happen to you.

The bad news is, the chemicals in conventional cleaning products can be toxic to you and especially dangerous to your developing baby. When you're cleaning, if the product you're using has a strong odor, of course you are breathing it in. It is entering your bloodstream, probably crossing the placenta—and chances are, it is toxic.

A tremendous amount of money and effort are spent each year to convince us to purchase all sorts of "special" cleaning products, some of which contain dangerous chemicals and even result in accidental poisoning. And the danger doesn't stop there. They wreak environmental damage when they are flushed down the toilet, poured down the drain, or tossed in the garbage. Now we know that they are actually unnecessary for getting your house "spic-and-span." In the case of cleaning, simple really is better. Simple products clean just as well, without any toxins to add to your (and your baby's) body burden.

WHEN CLEAN IS NOT GREEN
Ban the Bleach

One of the most common cleaning ingredients is also one of the most offensive. It can cause a host of problems including respiratory irritation, chemical burns, and immune disorders. Chlorine bleach is also the most common accidentally swallowed cleaning agent, and even a very small amount of it ingested can cause serious damage to tissues and organs and even death. Plus, bleach mixed with other common household cleaners, even vinegar, releases a highly toxic gas. So ban the bleach. Use hydrogen peroxide, baking soda, or vinegar instead.

Synthetic Fragrances

We covered phthalates in chapter 4. But the dangers of synthetic fragrances and phthalates are so big, and so relatively unknown, that they bear repeating. If something has a "springtime breeze" fragrance, or claims to be an "air freshener," remember, it is neither. Within the industry, these are called "masking fragrances," but just what are they masking? Usually they are added to products to cover up offensive-smelling chemicals. They also help hide the smell of whatever you're trying to clean up. But since chances are, you took out that cleaner to actually *clean* something and not just cover it up (heck, that's what that throw rug is for), you probably don't want to add one more layer to what is already there. Something clean should actually have no smell at all. So beware: Synthetic fragrances are lurking in almost every conceivable household product—and certainly in most of the "regular" brands. "Cleaning" solutions with synthetic scents are actually not so clean.

Remember: If a cleaning product has a synthetic scent, you should turn up your nose at it.

Corrosive Cleaners

Any corrosive cleaners should be totally off-limits, and not just when you are pregnant. Conventional oven cleaners and drain cleaners cut through all that thick gross stuff (baked-on grease or plugs of hair—blech!) by eating through it—chemically. They work by chemically melting, burning, dissolving. . . . You get the picture. They can cause chemical burns to the skin on contact and blindness if splashed in your eyes. These have no place in your home or life. (Might as well just put your head in the oven!)

Antibacterial: Good or Bad?

It sounds good, doesn't it? Aren't bacteria how we get lots of bothersome things like a sore throat or runny nose? Antibacterial add-ins seemed to appear in every conceivable product in the early 1990s: in dish-washing soaps, hand sanitizers, household cleaners, even in products for children. But at what cost? Almost immediately it became apparent that many users were experiencing unwanted side effects ranging from minor eczema and itching to serious dermatitis that could be cured with only steroid creams— something most experts would agree you do not want to use on young children, and certainly not on yourself if you are pregnant. Manufacturers responded by diluting the key ingredient in their antibacterial products. The reactions decreased, but they did not go away.

And that wasn't the only problem. The most prevalent active ingredient in antibacterial products is triclosan. There are highly conflicting studies on the safety of triclosan for humans and the environment. Some of those studies suggest that when triclosan is combined with the chlorine in tap water, it forms chloroform gas, which the EPA classifies as a "probable human carcinogen." In the UK in 2006, those findings prompted stores to pull hundreds of items from shelves for reformulating.

Not only is it unproven that antibacterial products clean any better than plain soap and water, but many experts believe we are playing a dangerous game with the delicate balance of "good" and "bad" bacteria here—that by using antibacterial additives in everything from room fresheners to dish soap, we are creating an army of supergerms. In other words, the bacteria that survive this constant onslaught are, of course, more and more resistant to the chemicals used to kill their weaker cousins.

WORD OF MOUTH Antibacterial additives are so widespread that you might not even know you are using them. They are in everything from over-the-counter acne medications to best-selling toothpastes and mouthwashes. Choose toothpastes like Desert Essence or Tom's of Maine. The Natural Dentist makes an incredible mouthwash that is not only triclosan free but that got my terrible pregnancy gingivitis under control—naturally! Beware of even trusted brands: Many toothpastes list triclosan as an active ingredient. You'll even find it added to plastics such as antimicrobial toothbrushes. 🍃

So are we doomed to constant, ineffective hand washing like Lady Macbeth? Out, out damned spot!

Not at all! You can clean yourself and smell good, and be gentle on the environment, too. Consider mild, tried-and-true basics such as Sappo Hill oatmeal and lavender handmade soap. I also love Vermont Soap Organics oatmeal soap—it's almost appealing enough to eat! (Don't, though. It doesn't really taste as good as it smells, as my seven-year-old will tell you. . . .)

To clean your home, choose all-natural products like the ones we discuss below. You can feel safe about what you're using, and I promise, this stuff really works!

Green Guru

Deirdre Imus

FOUNDER AND PRESIDENT, DEIRDRE IMUS ENVIRONMENTAL CENTER FOR PEDIATRIC ONCOLOGY
COFOUNDER AND CODIRECTOR, THE IMUS CATTLE RANCH FOR KIDS WITH CANCER
FOUNDER, GREENING THE CLEANING

OK, first just let me say this: No matter how healthy your self-esteem, you probably don't want to stand next to Deirdre Imus when you're pregnant. Or anytime within a year of giving birth. Oh, heck, maybe never! Her movie-star good looks combined with an athlete's body show, very clearly, that she won nature's lottery. And to top it off, she's a passionate powerhouse on a green mission of looking out for kids' health and well-being.

"Greening the Cleaning came out of working with kids at the Imus Ranch. We wanted everything at the ranch to be very healthy and nontoxic for these kids who were already sick, whose immune systems were compromised. Everything we used to build the ranch was nontoxic: no pressure-treated woods, no paints with VOCs. All of the food is one hundred percent organic. We have our own sustainable gardens and greenhouse. Everything for every meal is picked fresh daily. We don't serve meat or dairy, since these kids' bodies are already processing a lot. We're lucky because we've got a great chef there who can turn bok choy into something the kids say they love! The delicious food comes with a message: There's no reason not to start being healthy. It's never too late! Mothers need to have the confidence to say, 'I can do this for my family. Food can be good for them and good tasting!'

"Working with these kids inspired me to ask myself, if hospitals are healing places, shouldn't they be nontoxic? What can we do to make the cleaning cleaner? Hospitals do have germs and there are places that they need to use a germicide, but the most toxic cleaners were being way overused. They were used for everything, everywhere. And that just didn't make sense. We did the research. What you find when you look at the ingredients in those famous brands we all have (or had) under our kitchen sinks are things the EPA lists as known carcinogens, neurotoxins, probable human carcinogens, or poisons. Not things you want to use everywhere. So now hospitals and schools and other institutions that use our products limit the germicide to areas with certain needs, and Greening the Cleaning is doing its thorough, nontoxic cleaning job everywhere else.

"With the institutional line so successful, it was a natural move to the retail level. Our success comes from the fact that we have proved that our products

1. work as well or better than conventional brands,

2. are not just cost competitive but actually save money—between three percent and seventy-five percent,

3. contribute one hundred percent to charity—one hundred percent!"

Red Flag
chlorine bleach
drain cleaners
oven cleaners
petroleum-based furniture polish
conventional glass and countertop cleaners

CLEAN, GREEN HOUSE

The best household cleaners I know are probably already in your kitchen. They are tried-and-true and nontoxic—literally safe enough to eat—and as an added bonus, they're incredibly cheap!

Baking Soda

Baking soda is a gentle scrub to clean bathtubs and stainless-steel sinks. It is also the world's best deodorizer—and it does the job without any of those offensive "masking" fragrances. Plus it's terrific for washing the laundry. Yup, baking soda alone, about three-quarters of a cup for a big load, cleans everything from my husband's "aromatic" soccer gear to a toddler's favorite shirt. It's especially nice for bedding and towels; it makes them supersoft and doesn't leave behind waxy buildup or weird smells, as conventional detergent does. When I started using baking soda in lieu of laundry detergent, no one in my family even noticed, and my middle child's occasional rashes disappeared. Our clothes looked clean, smelled great, and felt nicer, too!

More ways to use baking soda:

• It is the best carpet deodorizer. Sprinkle it over a carpet, leave it for a couple of hours, then vacuum it away.

• Sprinkle it in garbage pails to absorb odors.

• Use it as a terrific bathtub scrub that won't scratch: Sprinkle some in the tub, then scrub with a clean rag or paper towel in a gentle, circular motion. Once spots are gone, turn on the shower and wash everything away. It's environmentally super friendly, so you won't feel guilty about passing it on to the frogs and fishies!

• Add a quarter to a half cup when you draw a bath to make a very, very soothing soak for minor skin irritations. It's safe for baby, too; just use much less, of course, as baby's bath is so much smaller.

- As you probably already know, baking soda is a safe, non-toxic tooth whitener. Put a little in your hand; dip in your moistened toothbrush to make a paste, and brush. The taste takes a bit of getting used to, though.

Vinegar

Vinegar is the ultimate all-purpose cleaner. (Well, it's good for *almost* all purposes: Do *not* use it on marble, which it can streak and stain!!!) It's incredibly green and super inexpensive. Dilute one part vinegar in four parts water to prevent streaks and staining. If you're turning up your nose at the idea of your house smelling like a salade niçoise, forget it. The smell evaporates when the vinegar dries.

Use it to clean the bathtub, toilet, and sink (it's especially effective coupled with baking soda). You can pour pure vinegar in the toilet bowl. It will help you easily brush away stains, and again, zero guilt for flushing it into Flipper's backyard.

Vinegar is the best glass cleaner in the world! Put the diluted mixture in a spray bottle (or a plant mister from a florist), then spritz and wipe as you would with a conventional cleaner. It also wipes through grease on stove tops, appliances, and nonmarble countertops.

Lemons

OK, lemons are a lot more expensive than baking soda or vinegar, but they certainly are nontoxic and they smell terrific. Plus, you'll love their cleaning capabilities:

- Mix a half cup of olive oil and a quarter cup of lemon juice to make a fab polish for wood furniture. Be careful with pianos, though: Don't get oil near the keys or pedals, as it can really disturb the tone.

• Send some lemon peels through the garbage disposal to take away even the stinkiest odors.

• As a chlorine-bleach alternative in a white wash, add a half cup of lemon juice with your baking soda. Only on whites, though, because it is a natural bleach!

If you don't want the bother of mixing your own cleaners, consider the safety and convenience of one of the super-natural brands.

The pioneer in the industry is Seventh Generation. The company's founder and owner, Jeffrey Hollender, changed his life and started his business after going through a serious asthma scare with one of his children. His child came through OK, but Jeffrey realized, in a deep and unforgettable way, that he could make a difference. The products that resulted are building a better world for our kids. Seventh Generation is a good choice for household staples like toilet paper and paper towels, too. Theirs are all chlorine free and recycled.

RAGS TO RICHES I must confess, I love paper towels. In fact, I have been known to actually get depressed when I'm down to that last eighth of a roll. (I'm not altogether evil, because I do buy Marcal or Seventh Generation, depending on which store I am shopping at. Both are one hundred percent recycled, so no tree guilt for me!) But a green friend convinced me paper towels are still consumptive and that rags are better (plus a whole lot cheaper) for many jobs. So I gave in and cut up three of my husband's totally antique tees and put them into domestic service. I drape them over the side of a bucket under the sink. If the cleanup is not too goopy, I rinse the rag in the sink and drape it again. If it's kinda grubby, I toss it directly into the bucket and when it's joined by a few of its friends, I run them through the wash. Now, here's a great incentive: Even if you shop around, a roll of good recycled paper towels will probably run you somewhere between a dollar thirty-five and two dollars a pop. And there's always a ton of stuff to be cleaned with a little one around, so I figure I probably save about fifteen bucks a month by using rags for half the cleanup jobs!

Green Flag
More clean lines I like:

- Ecover

- Deirdre Imus' Greening the Cleaning

- Begley's Best

- BabyGanics

Always be diligent in reading labels. Just like in the cosmetics industry, there is tremendous leniency on what manufacturers can claim is "safe" and "natural." Manufacturers are required to list only reactions associated with direct exposure, not long-term or cumulative effects. Anything that says DANGER or CAUTION doesn't belong in your hands when you're pregnant, or under your sink when baby arrives. (Just what does "Keep out of reach of children" mean when you've got it out from the cabinet and are spraying it on the kitchen table?)

Kevin Schwartz
FOUNDER AND VP, BABYGANICS

OK, so necessity is the mother of invention. But often dads get inspired by the little folks, too. And in the case of entrepreneur Kevin Schwartz, the cute little muse has four furry feet.

"My wife and I really started to build up an interest in natural cleaning because of a dog we adopted. He used to rest his chin on a glass coffee table in the living room. Well, he developed sore spots on his chin, and none of the vets we took him to knew what was wrong. One day we looked at him resting his chin on the coffee table and said, 'Maybe we should stop using that ammonia glass cleaner,' and of course he got better right away. We began to look at all the cleaning products in our home and I found out what those big bold words DANGER! WARNING! CAUTION! on the label mean. We had tried to eat healthy and lead a healthy lifestyle, and we realized our cleaning products were not helping us!

"When we decided to make BabyGanics, we knew we had to go all-natural, but really, we needed more than that. We wanted something that was one hundred percent safe to use: to breathe, to ingest, even to get into your eyes. Basically, we wanted products that were not harmful in any way.

"We worked with an experienced organic chemist to, first, determine the right set of safe and natural ingredients and, second, to make our products the most effective, so people would keep buying them. People often think natural cleaners are not as effective as conventional ones. But that's just not true anymore. The category has matured. There have been years of trial and error and experience, so now you can get really pure products that also work exceptionally well. That's what we always hear from our customers. They can't believe how well our stuff works!

"We made a conscious effort to keep everything simple. We make the four staples: all-purpose cleaner, glass cleaner, tub-and-tile, and floor cleaner. These will cover all your housecleaning jobs; you don't need a different product for every single chore. I don't know anyone who has room for all those bottles in a home with a new baby, anyway.

"Awareness is the key. Read and understand what's in a product, because if you are using it in your house, your child is exposed to it."

GREEN AT A GLANCE

Evergreen: Make your own cleaners from nontoxic ingredients, such as baking soda and lemons.

Pea green: Replace all your antibacterial hand soaps with safer basics like Dr. Bronner's or Sappo Hill. Use rags for some cleaning jobs.

Spring green: Stock your kitchen and bathroom cabinets with nontoxic cleaners, such as those made by Seventh Generation, BabyGanics, or Greening the Cleaning, and recycled paper towels and toilet paper.

Part II

Life with a Newborn: The Green Stork Delivers

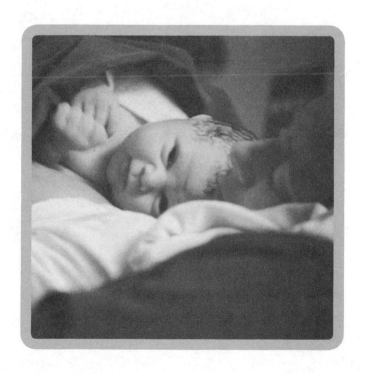

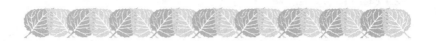

OK, your baby has made his entrance. He's the most charming, terrific, wonderful little person you'll ever meet. Also the most demanding, exasperating, dictatorial boss you'll ever have (maybe rivaling that one Fortune 500 CEO you once worked for . . .).

You'll want to give him everything he needs, because nothing in the world is too good for your wonderful baby.

Stores are built to house and sell the stuff you may want. Hundreds of millions of dollars are spent wooing your desire to fulfill his every need. (And assuage your every fear.)

What is actually any good? What do you need to be concerned about? What's worth your hard-earned dollars? And what will sit in the corner, mocking your waste of money and taking up valuable space?

This is really only the beginning of the decisions you'll be making for someone else. A very special someone.

I've put together some of the topics you may be thinking about for your home environment when baby is no longer in the secure domain of the womb. We'll look at how to help get baby the oohs and aahs she deserves from passersby when you're out on the town, and at the same time how to positively impact people on the other side of the world.

Hopefully, you or someone else in your household loves to cook, because you probably won't be frequenting the Russian Tea Room or Bouley quite as often now with junior in tow (they frown on slobbering patrons wearing bibs—unless they're very, very rich). We'll look at what you might want to whip up—and how to safely keep, freeze, reheat, and serve it, too.

And because your baby's circle of friends will be widening, our Green Gurus will give you tips to help convert even reluctant friends and relatives into your new Green Dream Team.

Seven

The Whole Kid and Caboodle

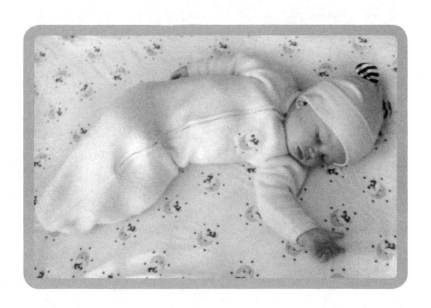

The Best Baby Gear

The image of a bright yellow rubber ducky bopping along in a ludicrously sudsy bath will forever be etched in my mind—beautifully at first, but now, like a good dream gone awry, fading first into trepidation, then advancing toward fear and finally anger.

Rubber Ducky, once a welcome member of the family, is now banned—it turns out that while masquerading as a friendly plaything, Rubber Ducky held some not so innocent secrets. In fact, Rubber Ducky wasn't really even rubber, after all. Rubber Ducky is made of polyvinyl chloride (PVC). PVC is a soft form of plastic that has now conclusively been proven to leach dangerous chemicals, including phthalates and bisphenol-A (BPA).

TOXIC TOYS

In December of 2006, the city of San Francisco sought to ban the sale of baby products containing certain potentially harmful chemicals. The ban was passed but was then halted, on appeal, pending further litigation.

The chemicals in question, phthalates and bisphenol-A, are in widespread use. And the most alarming news? They can be found in many items your baby may be using—and actively mouthing—every day: teething rings, soft plastic toys, and baby bottles.

Both phthalates and bisphenol-A are known endocrine disrupters, meaning they confuse normal hormone production, feminizing boys, and womanizing girls far earlier than normal. Hundreds of animal studies have linked phthalates to prostate and breast cancer.

What are these frightening substances doing in our babies' bottles and teething rings?

Consider the beginning of *The Graduate*, when Dustin Hoffman's future father-in-law whispers the secret to his terrific success: "I want to say one word to you, just one word. Are you listening? Plastics."

Today, as yesterday, there is a tremendous amount of money to be made, and a terrific amount of profit at stake, in the plastics industry. There is ensuing pressure in Washington and elsewhere to continue a climate of business as usual. According to *Time* magazine (Dec. 6, 2006), the American Chemistry Council says, "The crackdown on toys are [*sic*] not justified by the science."

Perhaps, but science has actually given us hundreds of animal studies that show damage to tissues and hormone reactions to these chemicals.

And common sense tells us a human study is hard to conduct and hard to fund.

Joel Tickner from the Lowell Center for Sustainable Production at the University of Massachusetts Lowell states in "A Review of the Availability of Plastic Substitutes for Soft PVC in Toys": "Scientists know very little about how the phthalates might affect a child's health, and direct evidence proving harm as a result of exposure to phthalates in soft PVC toys is impossible to obtain without conducting controlled experiments on children and looking for adverse effects throughout their lifetimes.

Acknowledging this, it is important to note that there are viable alternatives to soft PVC in toys. Why take a risk at the most critical stage in a child's development? Why focus on what a 'safe' level of phthalate exposure to a child might be, when this is fundamentally unknown? The terms of the debate, thus, must shift and focus not on how hazardous exposure to phthalates is but rather on whether there are safer substitutes for PVC and how these can be implemented."

As the *Time* story reports, "The *San Francisco Chronicle* recently had 16 toys tested in a private lab. One rubber ducky contained the phthalate DEHP at 13 times San Francisco's allowed level. A teether contained another phthalate at five times the limit. Meanwhile, a rattle, two waterproof books and a doll contained BPA, which is prohibited by the city at any level."

Given how bad the potential downside is, including reproductive defects and early onset of puberty, why are these products on the shelves of retailers we frequent, and trust? How do we know what's OK and what isn't?

Red Flag

soft squishy toys
anything that has a new-plasticky smell
vinyl washable baby books
most soft teethers, especially the water- or gel-filled kind
that can be put in the freezer

As with the ingredients in cosmetics, the U.S. does not require manufacturers to disclose ingredients in most nonfood consumer products, so until they do, we will have to be the watchdogs for our children's safety. Count on common sense: Is it super squishy?

Does it give off a chemical smell? If in doubt, just skip it. If babies are going to mouth it (and they will), better not opt for plastic at all if there is an alternative.

Fortunately there are now lots of new companies (and some old ones, too) making safer options available.

WOOD TO THE RESCUE!

For hundreds of years, parents have trusted teethers and toys made from wood. Now scientists have documented that wood has natural antibacterial properties.

Our own brand of baby rattles and wooden toddler toys, Earth to Kid (www.earthtokid.com), is made in Vermont and Maine and features baby-friendly finishes like beeswax.

Green Flag

I love the selection on these sites, too:

- www.rosiehippo.com

- www.plantoys.com

- www.monkeybeantoys.com

When you buy wood, however, please make sure it's domestic. Many wooden toys come from Thailand and China, where deforestation for cheap wood is taking a heavy toll. The environmental price goes up even more when you consider the long trip to the United States that those toys must make, and all the fuel that consumes. Also, beware of finishes and paints. If baby is going to mouth it, better go au naturel. Many other countries have much more "relaxed" policies concerning finishes on toys.

WIPES, LOTIONS, AND CREAMS

If you give birth to your baby in the hospital, as opposed to at home (or in a taxi, where I almost had my second), chances are, you will get a big package of free goodies delivered to your hospital room the day after delivery. It will likely be filled with disposable diapers, plastic baby bottles, hotel-sample-sized bottles of baby shampoo and lotion, and wipes, plus a pile of coupons for all the stuff you'll (supposedly) need to take care of baby.

Huge, multinational conglomerates pay a lot of money for the privilege of getting your attention during these amazing early days. The biological effects of your baby's birth have, quite literally, opened your mind. That open state is a survival-of-the-species gift from Mother Nature, who has endowed almost everything you see, touch, smell, and hear at this moment with special significance. Your brain is making synapses—connections—at a rate unheard of at any other point in your life, except when you yourself were a baby. Everything surrounding your baby seems imbued with this heightened importance—something aptly called the Halo Effect.

For you, that means what you already know: You won the lottery—this baby is special, thrilling, gorgeous . . . magnificent, actually. What it means to a marketer is that whatever you associate with your wonderful baby in these first few minutes, hours, and days will benefit from your powerful positive feelings, and will likely become a regular part of your life and your shopping list.

Unfortunately, lots of these products are not really so great, or the companies that make them wouldn't have to jump through such hoops to get them to you at this most wonderful but also susceptible time.

If you are well stocked before baby is born, you may just want to say no when the bag arrives, especially since most times it's a cheap waterproof vinyl tote that is meant to serve as a diaper bag. (Mine had a bad plasticky smell, which I now know meant it was putting out VOCs in my room!)

Skip the freebies and consider these very clean options:

Baby Shampoos, Lotions, and Oils
- Weleda Calendula Oil

- Burt's Bees Baby Bee Shampoo Bar

- Green Babies Organics Baby Me Shampoo and Tushy Tonic (our own brand)

- California Baby wash and shampoo

Baby Wipes
- Water and a soft cloth are just fine for the first few weeks, if you have the patience to run frequent washes.

- 365 baby wipes with aloe vera and vitamin E, from Whole Foods Market

- Seventh Generation baby wipes

- Tushies baby wipes

Don't forget: For anything you're using on baby, always check the ingredients list. Leave products with parabens and synthetic fragrances on the shelf! And please don't use any kind of powder or talc. Babies simply don't need it and the ensuing airborne particles are downright dangerous for baby to breathe in.

Green Guru

Dr. Lisa Ecklund-Flores
NEONATAL DEVELOPMENTAL PSYCHOLOGIST
FOUNDER AND DIRECTOR, THE CHURCH STREET SCHOOL
FOR MUSIC AND ART, MANHATTAN
PROFESSOR, MERCY COLLEGE
MOM

Dr. Ecklund-Flores has spent her entire adult life specializing in the joy and development of children. As founder and director of one of Manhattan's most applauded art and music schools, she would already have vast expertise. Add to that her work as a research scientist at the New York State Psychiatric Institute and her no-nonsense, makes-sense observations, and you can see why she is a sought-after speaker and consultant (including for *Blue's Clues*!).

"We are living in the golden age of information about child development. Advances in technology have made it possible to understand better than ever before what babies can do, and when they can do it. However, just because we discover something new about the way a baby sees, thinks, or learns doesn't mean that we have to buy something to make the baby 'better.' As a matter of fact, the very things that the baby biz pushes us to buy to make 'better babies' often do more damage than good.

"A prime example is the absurdity of fetal 'universities,' which use amplifying devices and stimulation routines. Not only do they fail to make mini-Mozarts, but they may actually impair the fetus' developing hearing and cause alarming physiological reactions. Sound is distorted in unpredictable ways in the fluid of the amniotic sac, and there is no scientific indication that bringing extra stimulation to the developing baby improves its well-being. The uterus is filled with low-frequency, low-intensity sounds, filtered by the natural buffer of the amniotic sac and tissues of the womb. No parent would blast loud sounds in the room of a sleeping newborn! Parents need to listen to their instincts and realize that playing loud sounds through speakers held up against pregnant mama's belly is just as ridiculous.

"Here's another example most everyone can relate to: Not long ago, researchers concluded that newborn babies best see contrasts of dark and light—rather than distinct colors and shapes. Fast on the heels of that information came the black-and-white nursery ensembles that many parents felt they had to buy: black-and-white mobiles, black-and-white comforters, black-and-white baby toys. The advertising message was that parents would promote better visual development in their newborns if they surrounded them with these items.

"Actually, newborns need the natural environment to promote normal visual development. They need the stimulation of the full spectrum of colors; they need to see their parents' facial expressions while they're being held and talked to. No black-and-white mobile is going to be as developmentally stimulating as watching your parents' faces as they talk to you. With Mom's and Dad's faces come their smells, their touch, and their voices—these are the natural 'organic' sources of sensory stimulation that are crucial to normal development.

"Countless videos and computer programs have been designed to make your baby 'better,' and parents are manipulated into believing that they are compromising their baby's potential if they don't buy these things. Parents have become the disenfranchised middlemen in their child's development, with advertising spin doctors interpreting developmental research in misleading ways in order to fabricate needs for their products.

"The bottom line is, you know what's best for your baby. In fact, you are what's best for your baby."

HOW WEARING BABY REDUCES STRESS, FOR YOU BOTH

A recent Columbia University study confirmed what many mothers instinctively know: Holding your baby has many benefits. It significantly lowers the stress hormone cortisol, and promotes mother-baby bonding. Indigenous cultures have long known about the benefits of baby wearing, a necessity in agricultural societies to keep baby safe while Mom worked the fields, tended the livestock, or went for water. Baby wearing has many benefits besides safety and convenience. There are many carriers on the market, but baby slings most closely duplicate the feeling baby had while still in the womb. Imagine how comforting it will be for baby to hear your sounds, smell your smell, feel the rhythm of your heartbeat, and be lulled by the gentle sway of being "worn" by you when you're walking. If that's not convincing enough, using a sling is way less hassle for you, too. It makes it easy to discreetly nurse, or snuggle baby while you're shopping or walking by gently adjusting the folds of the fabric. I loved using mine to carry all my kids, and some, like the New Native, are even available in organic cotton.

And if you think slings are just for crunchy granola eaters, think again. Cindy Crawford extolled the virtues of her New Native on *Good Morning America*. And such A-list supermoms as Angelina Jolie, Kate Hudson, and Rachel Weisz have been spotted toting their babes in them.

Slings aren't right for every baby, though. If you've got a kicker, a little tyke who pumps her legs all the time (preparing for the day she'll take off like Road Runner), she'll likely prefer a Baby-Björn or Snugli. These offer pretty good back support (and you may find you need it after hauling baby inside for nine months). And the real benefit is that baby can face in or out, depending on his mood or circumstances. My second baby, Mina, was a roly-poly little bowling ball for the first three months and loved her sling, but as soon as she could self-support her head, she wanted to see the world and preferred riding face out in her BabyBjörn. To me, this type of carrier is also the most secure-feeling.

Baby backpacks are the other option, and my husband preferred this (he said something about "a man's center of gravity"). Keep in mind, though, where you live and who will have access to baby in a backpack. Baby will be able to reach out for lots of things and will not be under your watchful eye back there, so backpacks may not be the best choice for crowded city environments.

Whichever you're considering, see if you can borrow one from a friend to try before buying, as all of these are fairly pricey, and you'll want to be sure you'll use it if you lay out the cash.

(An added bonus to baby wearing: Cortisol is often blamed for causing stubborn belly fat, and again, baby wearing is proven to reduce cortisol. So if you hold your baby, it might help you lose your spare tire—at the very least, it'll cover it up!)

SWEET DREAMIN', BABY

Unless you're choosing the family bed or otherwise cosleeping with baby, you're eventually going to need a crib mattress. Depending on what type of mattress you choose, this can be a fairly big expenditure. Regardless of how much you spend, though, it is a huge—potentially life-changing—decision. Babies and toddlers spend ten to fourteen hours a day sleeping and playing on a crib mattress. In oh-so-many ways, for oh-so-many days, the mattress is the single most prominent object in the child's environment. What you choose matters. So wake up, and look at what we've been sleeping on.

Over the last thirty years, natural crib-mattress materials have been replaced with inexpensive petroleum-based synthetics. Nearly all crib mattresses today contain polyurethane foam, vinyl (PVC), phthalates, chemical fire retardants, and an extensive list of added industrial chemicals.

There is growing concern among physicians, health professionals, public-safety officials, environmental-advocacy groups, and consumers regarding how these chemicals might affect our children. Many researchers suspect that toxic chemicals are playing a significant role in the dramatic increase in childhood disorders.

So, just because kids (and adults) have been sleeping on this chemical cocktail for years doesn't mean it's safe. Similarly, before it was found to be toxic and subsequently banned, lead paint was widely used and accepted as "safe." According to www.naturepedic.com, some researchers feel many components of today's baby mattresses are also toxic and, even though these chemicals are currently legal, believe they will eventually be banned, as well.

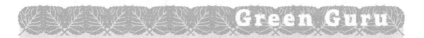

Green Guru

Barry Cik

FOUNDER, NATUREPEDIC

CHIEF ENGINEER, G.E.M. TESTING & ENGINEERING LABS

FATHER AND GRANDFATHER

Barry has a whole bunch of letters that follow his name and lots of mysterious but impressive titles including (feel free to skip ahead of this intro if, like me, you find his credentials make your head buzz) board-certified environmental engineer, qualified environmental professional, certified hazardous-materials manager, registered environmental manager, registered brownfield professional, forensic engineer, and registered professional engineer. Anyway, what this all really means is, he has the ways and means to know exactly what he is talking about—and it's important, so please don't skip this next part.

"When parents use a conventional crib mattress, the baby is, in a way, sleeping on gasoline. The foam is derived from petroleum. Companies need to dump a lot of chemicals onto that material to keep it from being highly combustible.

"The most common flame retardant used over the last several decades has been pentaBDE. Due to overwhelming evidence of its harmful nature, this chemical was banned in California as of 2006, and other states are following suit. It has also been banned by the European Union. Rather than panic parents, the U.S. government has not recalled all of the mattresses on the market—and in homes—made with pentaBDE. So if your baby is sleeping on a conventional crib mattress, she is probably sleeping on pentaBDE.

"If that isn't bad enough, some baby mattresses are being touted as 'antimicrobial' or 'antibacterial.' Manufacturers can make those claims when they add biocides, which are basically pesticides, to kill microbial life. But what are those biocide chemicals doing to the baby sleeping on that mattress?

"Four years ago, I was going to buy a mattress for my first grandchild. All of them were made with polyfoam and vinyl. I asked for other options and was told there weren't any. I did some research and found that there were, in fact, organic options. These were wonderful compared to foam, but they were basically tiny versions of organic mattresses for adults, and babies simply can't sleep on the same type of mattress we do.

"Here are the five basic problems with the natural/organic crib mattresses I saw:

1. **Ridges:** All had quilted or tufted surfaces, not firm, flat surfaces. You have to put an infant on a smooth surface. You don't want to risk the baby rolling over on her stomach and not being able to pick up her head. (In the United States,

sudden infant death syndrome is the number one killer of babies under twelve months.)

2. Wool: Wool isn't the right choice for infants, as many babies are allergic to wool.

3. Latex: Much latex is natural, but latex, too, is a very common allergen. There are currently more than a thousand pending lawsuits in U.S. courts dealing with babies and latex allergies.

4. Not waterproof: Natural is wonderful. But if you have a couple of accidents, the mattress will start growing bacteria. A good crib mattress has to be waterproof.

5. Poor surfacing: Dust mites are widely considered to be the most significant allergen there is. If you don't want to allow dust mites to grow on a baby's mattress, you must be able to wipe its surface clean.

"The bottom line: Don't put your baby on a conventional crib mattress. Choose one that's made with organic cotton instead of foam filling. Confirm that nontoxic materials such as food-grade polyethylene were used to make it water- and dust-mite proof and flame-retardant. (Of course, organic cotton is already safer than highly flammable petroleum-based foam.) Don't buy a baby mattress made from allergenic materials such as latex or wool. Finally, use a mattress with a firm inner spring and a flat, firm surface."

GREEN AT A GLANCE

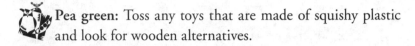**Evergreen:** Switch to a natural crib mattress and organic-cotton bedding.

Pea green: Toss any toys that are made of squishy plastic and look for wooden alternatives.

Spring green: Just say no to toys or gifts that don't fit your green philosophy.

Eight

Green
Jeans

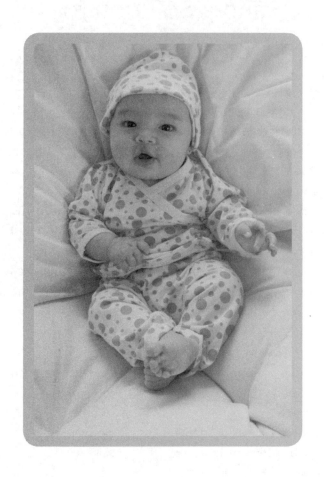

Coolest Organic Duds for Your Little Fashion Plates, and a Solution to the Diaper Dilemma

Babies need a seemingly mind-boggling amount of clothes. I couldn't even imagine mine would need what I saw listed on parenting sites. I assumed those were just plumped up to get you to buy more stuff, or meant for those lucky moms who could really splurge on swanky ensembles. But I was mistaken. These teeny-tiny people have lots of different liquids going in and out of their bodies (not always at the most convenient times). This means lots and lots of changes of clothing. And believe me, you do not want to be waiting on your dryer when junior needs fresh duds. So here's what you should probably have on hand when baby arrives:

THE OPTIMUM LAYETTE

1 take-me-home outfit

4–6 kimono sets or one-piece rompers

6 lap-over T-shirts or snappies

4–6 baby gowns or footy rompers

3–4 lightweight knit hats

4–6 blankets

4–6 bibs

2 cardigans

WHY ORGANIC MATTERS

I started Green Babies for my first child, and for yours. I had spent years as a model and had worn some of the coolest and finest clothes ever made. I knew something about how a great outfit can get you noticed and make you feel special. Because I started modeling at sixteen, by the time I had my first child at thirty, I didn't know too much about much else except, well, clothes. (OK, and how to order coffee and ask where the bathroom was in several different languages.) My husband had an amazing job in the arts in New York City, which meant lots of fulfilling work and long hours, but not a huge paycheck. We needed two incomes to survive. By tremendous good fortune, while I was sifting through the *New York Times* help-wanted ads (seeing all the great jobs I didn't have the skills or education for), I read a story about Texas farmers reverting to organic cotton farming, working the land as past generations had. I learned about the perils of conventional cotton—how, unbeknownst to most folks, this great American crop was causing sickness in farmworkers and devastating the agricultural landscape because of the amount of chemicals it guzzled. I had thought cotton was "the fabric of our lives." But I found out that conventional cotton was, in fact, the fabric of our lies.

I came to understand the firm conviction of the organic farmer, which is: Soil is an entire ecosystem of its own, filled with diverse living organisms that work in a harmonious cooperative that allows crops to grow. It is not dry, dead dirt that must be sprayed with toxic, petroleum-derived chemicals in order to produce commodities with no thought for the lasting destruction left behind.

In the early 1990s this way of thought was sweeping through the cotton fields of California and the high plains of Texas.

Third- and fourth-generation farmers, whose families depended on the crop for their livelihood, were converting back to organic, to the methods their grandfathers and great-grandfathers used, because of a deep love of the land and a belief that it was their responsibility to future generations.

This is the noble, natural start for the organic fibers that wind up on our babies' backs!

Before we let any fabric touch our babies' skin, we should ask ourselves:

- Where does it come from?

- Who made it?

- Who has touched it?

- Under what conditions was it made?

Big advertising agencies get paid a lot of money to help us forget to ask these questions! BUT IT IS IMPORTANT! How you feel about things—your values and beliefs—is important. Where your money goes and what happens to the planet are important! The quality of things, the intention behind the invention, are important! What your baby uses and smells and touches is important!

I have seen the curve with organic cotton, though it took much longer than I thought it would. For years and years I stood at farmers' markets and neighborhood festivals, sometimes in the pouring rain, selling rompers I screen-printed myself. I did nursery school fund-raisers. I walked around to stores with my kid in her sling and Green Babies samples in her diaper bag. I did craft fairs and street fairs the last days of both my second and third pregnancies. I put snaps in at the kitchen table. It took a long, long time of telling people over and over the difference organic cotton makes, and the change seemed to come about one garment at a time. And then, all of a sudden, in a blink, it hit the tipping point.

Now, almost fourteen years later, we are one of the fastest-growing brands of organic-cotton clothing in the world. And why not? Green Babies clothes are seen on the most beautiful and influential people in the world: babies.

Red Flag

Here are some of the things we've learned about conventional cotton:

- More energy is now used to produce synthetic fertilizers than to till, cultivate, and harvest all the crops in the United States.

- Conventional cotton covers only three percent of the world's farmland, but uses twenty-five percent of the world's chemical pesticides and fertilizers.

- In the United States alone, it is estimated, eight hundred million pounds of pesticides, herbicides, fertilizers, and chemical defoliants will be used on cotton this year!

- According to the EPA, seven of the top fifteen pesticides used on conventional U.S. cotton crops are potential or known human carcinogens.

- Some of the chemicals used on conventional cotton include the infamous defoliant paraquat and the insecticide parathion, which is sixty times more toxic than DDT.

Green Flag

With organic farming, crops are rotated to protect the soil, and farmers use compost and naturally derived mineral and plant products for fertilizer. Organic farming means the farmer lives in harmony with the soil and crops; he is cultivating life, instead of waging chemical warfare on his land.

Organic cotton makes for more than nice clothes; it makes for better lives.

A COTTON-PICKIN' SHAME

About four years ago, a study exploring the eradication of Third World debt stated that organic cotton was integral to getting Africa out of poverty.

In a natural farming cycle, a farmer grows his crops, sells some for profit, and saves seeds to plant the following year. But African farmers had come to rely on genetically modified seeds (GM: genetically modified; GE: genetically engineered; GMO: genetically modified organisms) bought from food giants. All needed synthetic pesticides and fertilizers; some were even genetically engineered to produce only sterile seeds. The natural cycle of "grow, sell, and save to replant" was broken and farmers were forced to use their profits to buy more seeds, pesticides, and fertilizers from the same food giants year after year. Like sharecroppers, the farmers remained impoverished as they grew crops that someone else would profit from.

These farmers also fell victim to what is known as "chemically dependent monocropping." Chemical giants peddled concoctions that promised higher yields and protection from predators. But those chemicals left the soil barren, and like a drug addict needing more and more to get the same high, the soil needed increased amounts of chemical fertilizers and pesticides in order to produce the same, or worse, results.

So it is with good reason that Tanzania, Ethiopia, and Uganda—among many other countries—have instituted government policies to enable many farmers to grow organic cotton. For the same reasons, humanitarians Bono and his wife, Ali Hewson, chose to use organic cotton for their world-changing, farmer-empowering, superchic Edun clothing line.

Manufacturers in the United Kingdom have eagerly embraced organic cotton. Many stores, including Marks & Spencer and Topshop, and many amazing designers, such as Katherine Hamnett and the artists at People Tree, have pushed organic cotton into the mainstream. Stores and designers in the United States have started a similar movement, and awareness of and interest in the huge difference organic cotton can make are growing.

If you're not feeling too weepy, visit www.ejfoundation.org, and check out the Environmental Justice Foundation's reports on the blanket poverty and devastation conventional cotton farming has brought to the nation of Uzbekistan.

AT LEAST WE DON'T EAT IT

Thank goodness for that, when you consider:

Between one and three percent of agricultural workers worldwide—that's between twenty-five million and seventy-seven million people—suffer from acute pesticide poisoning, with at least one million requiring hospitalization each year, according to a report prepared jointly for the Food & Agriculture Organization, the United Nations Environment Programme, and the World Health Organization. These figures point to acute symptoms of pesticide poisoning including headaches, vomiting, tremors, lack of coordination, difficulty breathing and respiratory depression, loss of consciousness, seizures, and death. Chronic effects of long-term pesticide exposure include impaired memory and concentration, disorientation, severe depression, and confusion.

A single drop of the pesticide aldicarb absorbed through the skin can kill an adult. Aldicarb is commonly used in cotton production; in 2003 almost one million kilos was applied to cotton grown in the US. Aldicarb is also applied to cotton in twenty-five other countries worldwide (source: ejfoundation.org).

So yeah, it's a good thing cotton isn't a crop that we eat. Can you pass me those potato chips/peanuts/cheese curls/insert favorite salty snack food here? Oh, wait a sec. What's that ingredient listed near the top? Hmmmnn, cottonseed oil . . .

BABY IS THE AMBASSADOR

Babies are celebrities in their worlds. They are welcomed with gifts even before they are born. Everyone wants to know what the baby's wearing, how she's sleeping, what the baby's eating. Strangers are charmed by baby's beguiling good looks. Schedules are changed around baby's wants. Babies deserve the best. They are filled with unlimited potential, and their arrival is the entryway to a better way for us all.

Because of what moms before you have chosen, the global market for organic cotton has increased twenty percent each of the past two years. Organic-cotton acreage in the United States expanded last year by eighteen percent. Supporting the American organic-cotton farmer is integral to "cleaning up our act" in so many matters-to-you ways. The EPA ranks the farming of conventional cotton as one of the top pollutants of our water and soil. Synthetic fertilizers, herbicides, and pesticides don't end up just on the leaves and fruit of the plants they're sprayed on. Any wildlife in the area—not just the bugs being targeted—are sprayed, too. Birds and animals eating the crops carry the chemicals in their systems, and literally pass them out the other end. But the most insidious pollution comes when the chemicals are washed off the plants by rain and irrigation and then seep into the groundwater. The EPA estimates that up to forty percent of the United States' groundwater, which is the drinking water for most Americans, is polluted with carcinogenic levels of pesticides from agricultural runoff.

Green Guru

Cliff Bingham
FOURTH-GENERATION ORGANIC-COTTON FARMER

Below, hear from a true American hero. Meet one of those cotton farmers in Texas who inspired me, by his courage and foresight, to start Green Babies:

"I started organic farming in 1992. The practice came from my philosophy: I don't consider myself an environmentalist, but a conservationist. The decisions I make are because I want to be a good steward to the land. And that means rotation of crops instead of monocropping.

"Capitalism is not a dirty word. I have heard the term Conscientious Capitalist, and I guess that's what I am. I'm not opposed to making money. But I think we need to be very careful of the decisions we make in this world.

"Last year, the yield on organic cotton was 3.3 bales per acre—over twice what I was doing in the 1980s, when my farm was conventional. Some of that is because the cottonseed breeders are pulling the strong seeds—no GM seeds, just strong cottonseeds—but part is because the soil is so fertile and healthy. About fifty-fifty, I'd say.

"Counting my son, who is already farming, we are five generations of farmers here on land my great-grandfather homesteaded. And it was basically organic until the fifties and sixties. They didn't call it organic back then, but that's what it was.

"Sustainability is not training farmers to plant cotton after cotton. It's just devastating to the soil. I've got eleven children, and I'd be a pretty rotten guy if I didn't have a game plan. I teach my children to be givers. You can be a giver and still be profitable.

"I got about twenty-five hundred acres here, and it's all organic. We work hard, but we love what we do."

COMMOTION IN THE OCEAN

One day when I was volunteering in a craft tent, making organic-cotton rag dolls with kids for Robert Kennedy Jr.'s Riverkeeper organization, I met a very smart young scientist who told me about the connection between conventional agriculture and the diminishing number of wild fish in the sea. Here's what she explained to me.

The same chemical fertilizers that are sometimes less than successful in growing crops on the farm (because the soil is depleted) have no problem doing their job on the pristine ocean floor of coastal waters. So even as chemical giants have failed to produce "super corn," underwater algae are growing to monstrous proportions. The overgrown algae strangle wild-fish eggs and raise the water's temperature by three or more degrees, making it a haven for jellyfish. Jellyfish also eat fish eggs. So it's a powerful double whammy. The "low" cost of conventional agriculture dramatically drives up the cost of wild-caught fish.

And the supposedly high cost of organic agriculture—which is not subsidized by the U.S. government—actually protects our land and the fruits of the sea.

ORGANIC FOR ONE HOT MAMA

Because people are starting to understand the huge difference buying and wearing organic cotton makes, there are now many cool clothing brands for women and men, too.

BRINGIN' ON THE GREEN

Who's got you covered in green? Try these labels:

- Good Karma Organics, one of our brands, www.goodkarmaorganics.com

- House of Hoss, a men's line by my husband, www.houseofhoss.com

- Stewart & Brown, www.stewartbrown.com

- People Tree, www.peopletree.co.uk

- Edun, www.edun.ie

- Wildlife Works, www.wildlifeworks.com

- Spiritex, www.spiritex.net

- Gaiam, www.gaiam.com

- Indigenous Designs, indigenousdesigns.com

And these cool online shops:

- www.cocosshoppe.com

- www.kaightnyc.com

If you're really looking for the greenest, swankiest haute couture and money is no object, check out Linda Loudermilk's line at www. lindaloudermilk.com.

Toni Pickette, a Los Angeles fashion stylist who has coordinated over five hundred fashion shows in her career, was the talk of Tinseltown recently with the "Think Vitality" show in Anaheim. "When they first came to me and said, 'We want you to style a full-scale fashion show and all the clothes have to be sustainable or organic,' I was a little worried," she recalls. "But it was an amazing experience. This show took the whole sustainable-clothing market to a new level. We're really seeing the craftsmanship from designers, with silhouettes that are chic and pretty. People can choose this and have trendy, high fashion. It's for anyone and everyone, not just the wholeheartedly environmentally committed."

Kathy Oglebay is the apparel specialist at Whole Foods Market's flagship store in Austin, Texas, and has a special perspective on the growth of this industry. "Organic-cotton apparel sales are growing rapidly," she says. "As people become more aware of its benefits to the environment and to their bodies, and the luxe feel of the fabric, they are seeking it out. Organic has appeal on so many levels: People want a better future and a safer place to live, and organic really speaks to that. Plus, it's great if you have skin conditions like eczema. The products have changed and expanded so much, even in the last two years. People often look at my clothes and say, 'That's organic?' They're surprised at how fashionable it is. It's very exciting to be part of this industry—to be part of the solution. The appeal of organic is vast, and quickly growing."

Green Guru

Vanessa Williams
ACTRESS, SINGER
MOM OF FOUR

The actress and singer Vanessa Williams is well-known for her profound talent, and is truly one of the most beautiful women in the world, inside and out—but few who don't know her would have guessed she's also an Earth Mother. . . .

"My first, Melanie, was born in 1987. I made a point to use cloth diapers; I didn't want to introduce any of the chemicals that might be in the disposables, and I wanted to be eco-minded. After six or seven months, though, I switched to disposables. They were just so much more convenient. In the world we live in, time is such a factor. Today there are much more eco-friendly options that allow mothers to be proactive about what they choose for their families and the environment. Cotton has always been my favorite fabric, for myself and my children. Now with so many options in organic cotton, a need is being filled: comfort for consumers and nourishment for the planet. We mothers now have choices that mean health for our families and other families, as well. I applaud the designers working with organic cotton.

"I was always into natural parenting. I breast-fed all my children. I made my own baby food, smashing those bananas in the kitchen. When I was growing up, we had our own garden. I grew up eating wonderful things like fresh tomato sandwiches. Living organically was always part of my life, a natural extension of who I am, and a great connection to happy memories."

THE DIAPER DILEMMA

Whether to wash or toss? This is a big decision. The right choice is different for every family. But whatever you ultimately decide, it's best to be fully informed about all your options. I can tell you I was no environmental angel. I went from evergreen to pea green to a pale-ish shade of spring green—not the direction I wanted to be going as a conscious consumer. But my humbling experience has made me something of an expert on all the possible options and their ramifications, both for your personal environment and for the world at large.

Here's how it went for me: My first baby, Layla, wore only cloth diapers, much to the dismay of my poor husband; our living room was frequently strung up with clotheslines of clean but slightly damp diapers, thanks to my environmentally sound but not-too-efficient Euro dryer. I tried to convince him we were doing our bit for the planet and that they looked artsy, a bit like Tibetan prayer flags. But it was pretty frustrating for him, so when baby number two, Mina, came along, we compromised: cloth diapers at home and Tushies (biodegradable and dioxin-free disposable diapers) for any urban jaunts. Baby number three, Nadia, never had the soft cush of fluffy cloth on her adorable tush. For her it was all Tushies, all the time. I told myself that at least they don't have that weird alien gel that expands diapers to six or eight times their original size. (Of course, this expansion continues in the dump. The gift that keeps on giving, the diaper that keeps on growing.)

The Dirt on Conventional Disposables

• Sixty percent of babies in the U.S. under twelve months get diaper rash.

• The rate of diaper rash increased from 7.1 percent of babies to 61 percent with the increased use of conventional disposable diapers.

• Sodium polyacrylate is the chemical that makes disposables superabsorbent—it can absorb up to one hundred times its weight in water. It can stick to baby's privates, and cause allergic reactions. In the U.S., this chemical was removed from tampons in 1985 when it was linked to toxic shock syndrome.

• Some studies show there is a rise in urinary-tract infections in babies as caregivers often change conventional gel-filled disposables less frequently than either cloth diapers or gel-free disposables, due to their superabsorbency.

• Superabsorbents also heat up when wet—a potential concern for boys' developing testes.

• Dioxin is a by-product of the paper-bleaching process used in manufacturing disposable diapers and is a carcinogen.

AT YOUR SERVICE?

Diaper service, that is.

Sorry, this one is not a green or toxin-free option, as I have yet to find a diaper service that does not use bleach (gallons and gallons of toxic bleach). This is very tough on the environment and not too soft on baby's skin, either. If you opt for cloth, better do them yourself.

As moms, we are juggling thousands of tasks and making hundreds of consumer choices every week. How we choose to diaper our wonderful babies has an impact on the environment. (Unless you join the few who—crazily? bravely?—opt not to diaper at all. But more on that later.) So it is important to keep our green perspective but also do what's right for our families. Here's a layman's look at how your options add up, dollarwise and earthwise:

Red Flag

Disposable diapers make up five percent of landfill waste in the United States. It can take up to five hundred years for a standard gel-filled disposable to decompose. The EPA estimates that about eighteen billion disposable diapers were discarded in America last year. The average American baby will go through five thousand diapers before graduating to the porcelain bowl, so your choice matters. And there are a lot of choices out there.

Green Flag

Here are some experts' perspectives on every one of them, from a more earth-friendly disposable all the way through a snazzed-up version of the age-old classic, cloth.

Green Guru

Jason Graham-Nye
OWNER, gDIAPERS

"My wife and I are from Australia. Four years ago, after our son, Flynn, was born, we were trying to cloth diaper when we came across gDiapers. We tried them and we just loved them. A gDiaper is a hybrid of cloth and disposable: a machine-washable cloth diaper cover with a snap-in liner. They're easier than cloth diapers, because rather than rinsing, you flush the disposable liner. They're less wasteful than disposable diapers, where you toss the whole diaper whenever you change.

"We were so passionate about using gDiapers that we bought the rights to manufacture and distribute them in the United States. gDiapers are better for baby and better for the planet. Disposable diapers were first manufactured in 1965. Before that, when the only option was cloth, about five percent of babies had diaper rash. Today, ninety-five percent of American babies are in disposables and about sixty percent have diaper rash.

"We hate the idea of all or nothing. Parents get so stuck on having the right system for everything from the moment the baby is born. We know so many cloth dropouts, and we think gDiapers are a good compromise. You just insert the disposable pad into the cloth cover and flush or toss it away when it's soiled."

gDiapers are easier on the planet because they create much less waste per change. However, they do use superabsorbent gel. So if you're looking for the convenience of a disposable that's also gel free, meet Green Guru number two:

Green Guru

Disposable-Diaper Pioneer Ed Reiss
CHAIRMAN, TUSHIES
FATHER AND GRANDFATHER

"My company started nineteen years ago. I was living in Sedona, Arizona, manufacturing plastic shoehorns. My baby daughter, Ilana, had terrible diaper rash. The doctors just couldn't get rid of it. I read a magazine ad for chemical-free, gel-free disposable diapers, and I ordered some. Within three days her rash went away. I said, 'If it's this good, I need to buy the company.' So I made a major lifestyle change and I was in the diaper business. Tender Care/Tushies was the first disposable diaper in the natural-products market. We have always been the leader in chemical-free diapers.

"We've always been gel free and chlorine free. Now we use a blend of wood pulp and cotton for the fill. It does the job and doesn't put chemicals against baby's tender skin.

"We've diapered tens of thousands of babies. I have three kids and three grandkids. They are all Tushies babies. Love is a great motivator."

If you are even thinking about going partly or all cloth, let your fingers do the walking over to www.tinytush.com. This family-run business is a veritable Wikipedia of all things soft and cloth for your baby's bottom. Owner and founder Charlene Foster has diapered a whole lotta bottoms: She has five kids, ranging in age from twenty-two to seven. She and her husband live on a forty-acre organic farm that grows produce and free-range organic meats and fowl. (If that all makes you feel a little inferior, fear not—Charlene is no holier-than-thou green queen.)

Green Guru

Charlene Foster

OWNER, TINY TUSH CLOTH-DIAPER BUSINESS
MOTHER OF FIVE

"The only child I exclusively cloth diapered was my youngest. I found the standard three-fold diapers frustrating. They were labor-intensive and not absorbent enough. I was doing way too much laundry because of leaks and accidents. If a system's not working, you just can't stick with it. I tried a lot of different diapers, but I didn't find any I thought were perfect. So I started tinkering with what was out there and came up with the Tiny Tush All in One. Cloth diapering is growing because of knowledge.

"Cloth is better because you have no chemicals against baby's sensitive skin, you have natural breathable fabric, and it's really tried-and-true—people have been cloth diapering for centuries. The Internet makes it easy. We can offer so many more choices than a grocery store or a department store.

"Every family thinking of cloth wants it for different reasons. They might be concerned about the environment, looking to save money, or have a baby with sensitive skin. Cloth diapering is right for any of those reasons, and a natural choice if you have the right tools.

"The Tiny Tush biodegradable liners make cleaning up cloth diapers easy. It's a thin sheet that keeps solids from sticking to the cloth diaper (and believe me, it can be sticky . . .). They take the 'Yuck!' out of cloth diapering; there's no dunking or soaking soiled diapers. Just remove the soiled liner and flush it away, then launder the diaper."

A BIG MOVEMENT (I COULDN'T RESIST!): *NO DIAPERS AT ALL*

If you have time, patience, and a big backyard, diaper-free devotees say you can save thousands of dollars, avoid diaper rash, and of course save landfill space by going without diapers, even from birth. (This is a concept my Mina highly advocated as a baby. She would strip down to nothing at any and every occasion, especially if she heard a song she liked. She would take off her pants and her diaper and do a wiggle dance!) If you're interested in exploring this zero-landfill option, check out the book *Diaper Free* by Ingrid Bauer.

GREEN AT A GLANCE

Evergreen: Pick your cotton carefully. Choose organic cotton whenever possible for you and your baby.

Pea green: Change the world, one diaper at a time. Go cloth when you can, even if it's just occasionally.

Spring green: Be especially suspect of inexpensive cotton clothes from Third World countries. The store you bought them from is making a profit, and so is the shipper, so if it seems too good to be true, someone, somewhere, is probably not getting a fair deal.

Nine

Home Environment

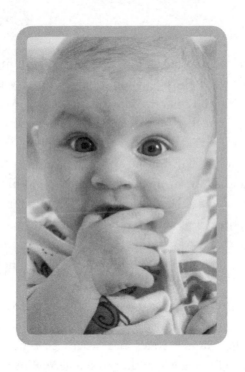

How to Detox Your Nest Without a Huge Overhaul

Whether you rent or own, whether it's a rambling old farmhouse or a high-rise condo, you've probably put a lot of thought, effort, and money into your abode. And certainly "home, sweet home" takes on even greater significance when you have a baby. Home is a refuge, a place to lay your weary head and recharge for another day. But just how sweet is your home?

Children and adults in the United States spend ninety percent of their time indoors. The EPA estimates that indoor air is two to seven times more polluted than outdoor air—and way more than that in homes that use air fresheners.

The number one trigger of childhood asthma is indoor air pollution.

You might think, "That's bad, but it won't affect me." Well, the odds are in your favor, but they're not great. One out of seven children in the United States has what's classified as chronic asthma. And pediatricians say that's a staggering increase over the numbers from just ten and fifteen years ago.

CAN THE BUG SPRAY
The best gift you can give your baby and your family (and yourself!) is getting rid of any pesticides you have around the house,

and never purchasing or using them again. Childhood cancer and leukemia are on the rise, and many cases are attributed to "environmental" causes. Just what does that actually mean?

Numerous studies have linked the use of "off-the-supermarket-shelf" bug sprays and foggers to childhood brain cancer and leukemia. Even back in 1987 a study in *Journal of the National Cancer Institute* determined that children exposed to pesticides in the home or garden were three to six times more likely to contract nongenetic leukemia than children who were not exposed. The stats haven't changed since, and it's not only cancer. A recent study published in *Environmental Health Perspectives* has found a link between POPs (persistent organic pollutants, which include some pesticides) and diabetes. Numerous studies cite a link between pesticide exposure and the later onset of Parkinson's disease. Although many factors may contribute to these diseases, reducing substantial risks certainly makes sense.

You might assume that the products on the shelf at your local drugstore or supermarket are safe. Surely companies wouldn't be allowed to sell them otherwise, right? But mounting scientific and medical evidence shows that might not be so. Take the case of DEET, a chemical in many brands of insect repellent. Only a few years ago DEET was considered "safe"; it has now been implicated in the serious health problems—and possibly even the deaths—of countless children.

Lab tests on animals at Duke University have revealed that frequent and prolonged exposure to DEET causes serious brain-cell death and behavioral changes. The researchers warn, "Use DEET with caution, especially [on] children, who are more vulnerable to brain defects that prolonged exposure to DEET causes."

Further research could show similar dire effects of other pesticides.

This doesn't mean you're doomed to be mosquito food. *Consumer Reports* found lemon eucalyptus oil to be about as effective as repellents containing DEET. And Australians, who live with what may be the biggest, baddest bugs on the planet, swear by tea tree oil, which is good for pets, too. (Tea tree oil is not recommended for infants, though; while it's natural, it can mimic estrogen.)

HOME SICK HOME

When the label on an oily spray that is a pesticide says, "Keep out of reach of children," what does that really mean? How far "out of reach" is an oil you use on your kitchen counters or floor? I remember reading that if you had a perfectly even surface, an ounce of oil could be spread some ridiculous distance—one square mile, I think.

Remember, the EPA tells us, "There is no safe level of pesticides"; there are just levels that pose a "lower risk." But of course, when the "risk" is childhood cancer, "lower" is probably not low enough.

Tessa Hill, who runs the educational nonprofit Kids for Saving Earth, paid the highest price, and doesn't want other parents to do the same. "I grew up in Minnesota and had never seen a roach," she says. "When I moved to Texas, I encountered roaches and learned that four times a year, everyone sprayed their houses with pesticides. Our dog also got fleas, so we used flea powder. Then my ten-year-old son, Clinton, came home from school with head lice and the school nurse insisted that I use a pesticide-based lice shampoo." Six months later, Clint was diagnosed with a brain tumor. Before he died at age eleven, he started Kids for Saving Earth because he wanted to keep our world, and the kids in it, healthy. "I want people to know that there are safe ways to get rid of bugs," Tessa says.

Recent studies suggest links between common amounts of pesticide exposure and a host of other problems, including low birth weight, aggressive behavior, impaired motor function, and ADD and ADHD.

Here's the good news: You're not doomed to a lifetime of living with creepy-crawlies. There are natural and effective means of controlling pests without resorting to out-and-out "combat." Because, after all, who wants to wage chemical warfare in her kitchen?

Here's a comprehensive plan from Beyond Pesticides to prevent or put a stop to whatever is bugging you:

PREVENTION
Structural

- Caulk, weather-strip, and repair any holes larger than one-sixteenth of an inch around water pipes, baseboards, electric fixtures, outlets, light switches, doors, and windows.

- Screen over windows, vents, floor and sink drains, and ducts.

- Keep trash, leaf piles, and woodpiles away from your home.

- Fix leaky faucets and drains.

- Insulate pipes to prevent condensation.

Cultural

- Discard newspapers, magazines, and paper bags.

- Inspect all food brought into your home.

- Store food in tightly sealed containers or in the refrigerator and put pet food away overnight.

- Clean all spills immediately.

- Wipe all counters and tables after use.

- Keep the stove grease- and food-free.

- Rinse food and drink containers before you throw them away.

- Empty trash and recycling bin frequently.

- Use trash cans with tight-fitting lids and avoid placing them under sinks.

- Avoid soaking dishes overnight. Always wipe the sink dry before leaving the kitchen for the night. Place sponges and dishrags in an airtight container.

- Don't overwater plants.

Monitor

- Once a month, place two sticky traps in each room roaches might travel through. (Put them where the floor meets the wall or countertop, inside cupboards, under the sink, and behind appliances.) Leave them for twenty-four hours, then discard.

CHUCK THE CHOOS AND BAN THE BLAHNIKS!

Well, OK, don't really chuck your Choos (unless you're a size 8½, then you can send them to me), but do consider leaving your shoes at the door. Did you ever stop to think where the soles of your shoes have been and what could be on them? And I don't mean just the usual dirt and occasional gross-o piece of chewed Juicy Fruit. "There's a lot packed into your shoe treads," says

Christopher Gavigan, executive director of Healthy Child Healthy World. "Microscopic pollen and soot particles, when tracked inside, can waft up into our eyes, throats, and noses. By taking off your shoes, you're preventing toxins from getting into your baby's system."

Green Guru

Kimberly Fusaro
WRITER, FASHION TRADE AND MAJOR WOMEN'S LIFESTYLE MAGAZINES

Kimberly has compiled some compelling reasons why you want to be a shoe-free devotee, too.

"Even if your shoes look clean, there's plenty of dirty stuff you can't see. Researchers from the University of Southern California found DDT in the carpets of almost a third of the homes they visited—twenty years after DDT was banned.

"It's not only what's on the bottom of your shoes that's dangerous; what's on top can be nasty, too. Waterproofing sprays and shoe polishes are highly toxic and have been known to cause serious allergic reactions.

"Make your home a haven. In many cultures it's a sign of respect and spirituality to remove your shoes. Think of the pagodas in Japan or the monasteries in Sri Lanka. Plus, removing your shoes will preserve your flooring and carpets.

"Offer guests cuddly socks or slippers at the door; they'll

probably take the hint and you won't have to bother explaining your philosophy. To go super green, pick up a few pairs of TOMS shoes (www.tomsshoes.com) in common sizes and leave them in your foyer for guests to use when they're inside your home. They're super comfy, and for every pair you buy, TOMS Shoes will donate a pair of new shoes to kids in need.

"For workmen who do not want to take off their protective boots, keep a box of inexpensive ShuBee shoe covers (www.shubee.com) at the door. They're just like the ones surgeons wear in operating rooms, and can easily be pulled over their boots, so whatever is on the bottom of their boots won't get pulled through your door."

GROW IT CLEAN

In the hit musical *Little Shop of Horrors*, sweet and mild-mannered Seymour works in a florist's shop. He has a host of problems, and only one friend, a mysterious and very large Venus flytrap he calls Audrey II. In return for good care and constant feeding, Audrey II promises to get rid of all of Seymour's problems, and she does—she devours them! If you choose them carefully, your houseplants will do the same for you: They will destroy your enemies.

NASA PUTS MAN ON MOON AND SOLVES INDOOR AIR POLLUTION PROBLEM *(NO, REALLY!)*

NASA announced the findings of a two-year study that suggests that common indoor plants may naturally combat indoor air pollution by removing several key pollutants. "Plants take substances out of the air through the tiny openings in their leaves," a NASA researcher says. "Research in our laboratories has determined that plant leaves, roots, and soil bacteria are all important in removing trace levels of toxic vapors."

These ten plants are the most effective, all around, in counteracting off-gassed chemicals and contributing to balanced internal humidity:

Areca palm	English ivy
Reed palm	Australian sword fern
Dwarf date palm	Peace lily
Boston fern	Rubber plant
Janet Craig dracaena	Weeping fig

Some can be toxic if ingested, so keep them out of reach of children and pets. For more information, check out www.mont gomerycountymd.gov/content/dep/greenman/cleanairplants.pdf.

While you're there, note the other toxic bulbs and blooms (even beauties like azaleas can be poisonous).

Green Guru

Christopher Gavigan
EXECUTIVE DIRECTOR AND CEO,
HEALTHY CHILD HEALTHY WORLD

Here are a few more simple steps to "clean up your indoor act." The biggest and easiest-to-navigate clearinghouse for information on this subject is Healthy Child Healthy World, an organization that has tirelessly worked in the fields of science, medicine, and media to get the word out on how to protect our kids.

"It's all about simplicity and knowing the good choices. Healthy Child does the due diligence to make those choices easy and clear for parents.

"For more than sixteen years our former incarnation, the Children's Health Environmental Coalition, was a national leader in protecting children. In the beginning it was all about gathering the data and setting legislation. We were instrumental in working with Senator Barbara Boxer on the Healthy Schools Project. We were gathering the credible science and research that helped fund and support groundbreaking studies like 'The State of Children's Health and Environment' with John Wargo at Yale. Now we've expanded our focus to be a hands-on resource for parents, and to clarify our new role, we changed our name from CHEC to Healthy Child Healthy World.

"We are living in a very special time. Many more enlightened businesses are launching with our children's health in mind; our role here is to sift through them to find the real deal, so your job as a parent is easier.

"Every family has an impact on larger issues: global warming, deforestation, overfishing, soil erosion. What you do in your home radiates out to the world, and it begins with the tiniest and most valuable footprint, your child's.

"There are five easy steps we all can take to prevent harm and improve our families' lives:

Step 1: Avoid use of all pesticides and insecticides.

Step 2: Use nontoxic or natural household cleaners and products.

Step 3: Clean up indoor air.

Step 4: Eat more organic food.

Step 5: Use plastic products wisely."

Green Guru

Marie Myung-Ok Lee

PROFESSOR, BROWN UNIVERSITY

FOUNDER, GREENFERTILITY. BLOGSPOT.COM

MOTHER

When I met Marie she was a whirling dervish, just finishing her book tour for her best-selling *Somebody's Daughter*, researching a piece she was doing for super-green Web site treehugger. com, and beginning work on her next book, a study of autism. She really opened my eyes to how devastating environmental toxins can be to children and the people who love them.

"Six years ago, our then-eighteen-month-old, Jason, was diagnosed with a rare kind of neural tumor that was dangerously large and growing right on his spinal cord. A year later, he was diagnosed with another dire neurological problem: autism.

"During this time, I began researching intensively. My husband and I have no family history of neural cancers, or anything even vaguely resembling autistic disorders. I got to wondering whether there might be something from the outside, perhaps in the environment, affecting our son. We already ate and lived organic, but one thing my research on neural cancers and autism (and ADHD and related neural problems) kept coming back to was heavy metals. My mother had had a bunch of mercury dental fillings put in rather messily and haphazardly by our small-town dentist (after a car accident) when she was in her first trimester, pregnant with me. And I went on to have a bunch of mercury-containing vaccines when I went to Korea to research my novel, shortly before I conceived my son. I also got a mercury-containing flu shot when pregnant.

"Many heavy metals are extremely toxic to the human neural system, as evidenced by the expression 'mad as a hatter.' (In olden times, hatters used mercury to cure the felt they used and were vulnerable to mercury poisoning; symptoms included tremors and twitches, confused speech, even hallucinations and psychosis.) The unborn fetus can be particularly vulnerable to these kinds of toxic assaults, as heavy metals are not screened out by the placenta.

"The reason heavy metals are so ubiquitous is that (as the hat manufacturers knew) they are useful in industrial processes. Lead is a great 'fixer.' It keeps PVC plastics and glazes from chipping, and did the same when it was used as additive in paint. Mercury is an antimicrobial—it kills microbes, but it also kills neurons. Aluminum is light and easily malleable. Because toxic heavy metals are so very useful, you might find arsenic in your crib mattress, mercury in your flu vaccine, and aluminum in your antiperspirant. You might find lead in the balsamic vinegar on your salad, in the dirt outside your home, and even in the wires of your Christmas lights!

"So you see, the bad news is heavy metals lurk everywhere. We know they are toxic, but we really do not know how intensely they harm us, or how much exposure is too much.

"The good news is there are many simple and effective things you can do to minimize your baby's exposure:

• If you live in a house that was built before 1978, have the paint checked by a home inspector. Have the water checked, too, if you have lead pipes. Before filling baby's bath, run the hot water for a minute or two to flush out the water in the pipes that's been sitting there, possibly absorbing metals.

• Replace mercury thermometers with digital ones. Dispose of mercury thermometers safely—the mercury in one thermometer can contaminate a lake—by calling your local hazardous-waste disposal service. (Sometimes they'll give you a new thermometer for free!)

• Avoid using PVC plastics, especially in containers that will come in contact with food. Replace your vinyl lunch bag with one made from cloth or paper.

• Don't cook in aluminum foil, especially foods that are acidic or are being cooked at high heat, such as roasts. Store foods in glass containers or wax bags rather than tin foil.

• 'Silver' dental fillings are made, in part, from mercury. It's a good idea to avoid the dentist's office while you're pregnant or breast-feeding, but if you must have dental work done, request porcelain or composite ('white') fillings. This is NOT the time to replace your mercury fillings; disrupting mercury fillings and having mercury moved around in your mouth can cause your body to reabsorb it.

• Avoid fish higher up on the food chain, including tuna, tilefish, swordfish; little fish absorb some mercury, but the big fish that eat them are contaminated at much higher levels. If you're eating fish just for the beneficial omega-3 fatty acids, instead take a good fish-oil supplement that is either distilled or tested to ensure it is free of heavy metals.

• Switch to a natural deodorant; antiperspirants rely on aluminum-based compounds that swell the sweat gland shut.

• Don't 'pass on' antique hand-painted toys or furniture. If Grandma insists on giving them to you, try putting them in a place of honor (like a glass case!) where baby will not have contact with them.

• A vacuum with a HEPA *[high-efficiency particulate air]* filter will suck up metal-contaminated dust and not spit it back into your air.

• Insist on thimerosal-free vaccines for yourself and your baby.

"Now, after making more organic choices and eliminating (as best we can) sources of heavy metals and other toxins, I'm proud to report that our son has passed the magic five-year mark for being tumor free, and his overall health (and mine as well) is markedly improved.

"You don't need to experience a medical catastrophe like we did in order to start thinking in a new way. Know this: Clean, green, and natural is best. Even so-called 'safe' amounts of toxins can add up, especially when they interact with each other in unpredictable ways."

CLEAN SWEEP

You probably tossed the nail-polish remover and drain cleaner before baby was born. But take another look around your house—in the back of the cabinets and under the bed—to see what might be lurking there, because if baby's not on the prowl yet, she soon will be.

Of course you need to gate stairs, lock toilets, plug outlets, wind up cords on your blinds, and encase any electrical cords, too. If you have baby in a crib, drop down the mattress to the lower position before he can pull up. I strongly suggest gating off the kitchen so you can actually (occasionally at least) make something hot to eat.

If you have the resources, you may want to hire a professional baby-proofer. The work will be done in a day. She'll bring all of the supplies, and she may save you and your mate from several rows. Baby-proofers buy their goods at wholesale, so hiring one may save you money, too. They won't go through your drawers, though, or sweep under your bed (darn it!), so here are steps you'll need to take yourself on your clean, green sweep:

• Dump just about everything stored under the sink. Toxic household cleaners, bug killers, bleach. Dispose of these products properly, not by pouring them down the drain (your local municipality will have toxic-item pickup days or drop-off locations).

• Vacuum under the beds and other furniture to remove dust mites. A vacuum with a HEPA filter is the best.

• Give everything metal—including drawer pulls—a second look. About seventy percent of drawer pulls contain potentially dangerous levels of lead. Unfortunately you're probably not going to be able to tell if the metal in your drawer pulls contains lead; even those that look like brass are typically made from metal compounds. Unless you specifically know something is lead free, consider replacing it.

• Pull change and small objects out of the backs of drawers and pack them away safely. As soon as baby can pull up, he has access to whatever is inside. Go through the backs of linen closets and medicine cabinets, too.

• As a general rule: If you don't want baby to eat it, play with it, or find it (and she will), don't bring it into the house.

• Double-check to ensure that all medicines are in child-proof containers.

• Throw away anything with synthetic fragrances, including cosmetics, cleaners, solvents, and air fresheners. Even very young children are conditioned to think if it smells good, it'll taste good, too.

• One more time: Get rid of pesticides (remember that little fingers can easily reach into ant and roach traps), chlorine bleach, caustic drain and toilet cleaners, and rubbing alcohol. My youngest daughter took a huge swig of rubbing alcohol and we had three paramedics on our front lawn five minutes later. She was fine, but we were lucky. (And dumb.)

BUILDING YOUR GREEN HOUSE

Families welcoming new babies often need to move to a bigger home or remodel their existing one, but there are several precautions you need to take before starting construction. Many building materials are dangerous for pregnant moms and new babies. Here are some problems you might encounter:

• **Asbestos.** If your home was built before 1978, chances are, it has asbestos somewhere in the insulation. Undisturbed asbestos is like a sleeping bear: It probably won't harm you if you leave it completely alone, but you better be ready to run if you poke it! If you're going to have any demolition done, be sure to have someone experienced in asbestos removal check it out and institute the correct procedure. And don't plan on staying in the house while the work is done.

• **Lead.** As with asbestos, a house built before 1978 probably has lead paint somewhere in the interior. You'll want to test for lead before you move in or make any remodeling decisions, especially if you'll be doing a lot of sanding, which can spread lead dust everywhere. Removing wallpaper can be a problem, too, because it can expose old lead paints underneath. Better just leave that grandmotherly floral alone (think Martha Stewart) or have it painted over. For lead tests, visit www.leadinspector.com.

• **Paint.** If you decide you need new paint, don't do it yourself, even with a mask, and don't stay in the house while it's being done. Allow plenty of ventilation time for the paint to off-gas before you or your family members return. Choose a water-based paint with no or low VOCs. As a general rule, the shinier the paint, the higher the level of VOCs. Shop around: Even big-chain hardware stores, such as Home Depot, now offer greener options. To find superclean paint, visit www.AFMsafecoat.com.

• **Floors.** Besides the crib mattress, the floor is where your baby will spend most of his time. Don't go for wall-to-wall carpeting; regular carpeting gives off a number of VOCs. Carpets are one of the most toxic off-gassers there are, plus they're incredibly hard to keep clean. And as baby learns to roll, crawl, and cruise, she'll be pulling out fistfuls and mouthing it all the time. If you want padding by the crib in case of a tumble, consider a natural-fiber area rug. If you need to lay new tile, the greenest options are those made with ceramic or stone. Poured concrete is also easy on the environment and safe for baby.

Those seductively easy-to-peel-and-apply vinyl floor tiles are not a good choice, either. (I used them on my kitchen before I knew.) Not only does the adhesive backing have toxins, but the tiles themselves are filled with phthalates. If your kitchen or bathroom is already vinyl tiled, it's probably best to just leave it be. When you clean the tiles, don't use any harsh solutions or you'll risk breaking down the soft plasticizers, which will end up in your air. Never, ever use a product containing bleach on vinyl flooring; the combination of bleach and vinyl can create a very toxic chemical compound.

Bamboo flooring, one of the greenest options, can be found just about everywhere now. It is more expensive than wooden floors, but not much more. You can even get it at IKEA. If you choose bamboo floors, choose a shoe-free home, too. Bamboo is not as durable as hardwood.

Green Guru

Jesse Johnson
COFOUNDER, Q COLLECTION ·

Of all the green purchases you may be making, the crib, bassinet, or cosleeper you choose might be one of the most significant. Jesse Johnson of Q Collection makes furniture that is better for you, your home, and our planet. Q Collection is made from forestry-certified woods and formaldehyde-free, biodegradable textiles, and is so stunningly designed that it's been lauded by *Town & Country*, *Time*, the *New York Times*, and *California Home & Design*. And here's the really good news—the company recently launched Q Junior, an upscale but not astronomically priced collection just for the young-uns.

"Design, quality, and sustainability are what matter to us. In every product we make, we consider health and the environment. We use water-based nontoxic finishes and earth- and people-friendly fabrics, such as viscose, wool, organic cotton, and alpaca. All of our cribs are made by hand by craftsmen and -women here in the United States.

"When you're looking for furniture, consider these guidelines to help you make a sustainable choice:

• Choose furniture made from U.S. wood. Furniture that is created locally is only shipped a few hundred miles, instead of being shipped across an ocean.

• Support domestic craftsmen who have been doing this work for generations.

• Choose FFC-certified wood. All wood is not created equal. The U.S. imports more threatened tropical hardwoods than any other nation in the world. The conventional-furniture industry is one of the prime culprits.

• Look for GREENGUARD certification, which guarantees the wood won't interfere with indoor air quality."

GREEN AT A GLANCE

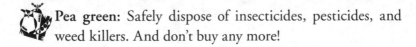 **Evergreen:** Hang wool rugs on the clothesline (just stay on the lookout for animals and rain) to really send mites running. Air out new carpets the same way. Put newly delivered furniture outside for at least a few hours, so it can off-gas in the backyard, not in your home.

Pea green: Safely dispose of insecticides, pesticides, and weed killers. And don't buy any more!

Spring green: Clean the filter in your air conditioner. It will work more efficiently, which will save you some cash, and improve your indoor air quality. Better yet, open your windows wide, which can reduce indoor pollution up to fifty percent. Always let the sunshine in! Dust mites can't stand sunshine.

Ten 🍃
The Age of
Asparagus

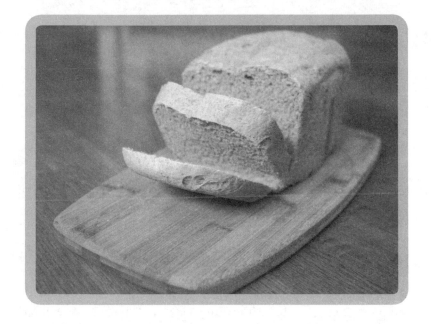

Getting Your Kitchen Top-Drawer for Your Fab Family

I never thought I'd spend a lot of time in the kitchen. My mother didn't like to cook, so we ordered in a lot when I was growing up. When I was modeling, most meals consisted of a cappuccino, or if I was really, really hungry, two cappuccinos and a piece of fruit.

When I became pregnant with Layla, I ate whenever I was hungry, but my husband and I were still going to restaurants a lot, or I was grabbing a quick bite while I was out and about, so I still didn't really plan meals or cook. Basically, I didn't have to think about feeding anyone but myself.

But when baby number one entered the picture, I was home a lot more. Chances are you will be, too. Whether you are working outside the house or not, many more of your meals will be consumed at home, even before baby is eating solids. And those meals will be more important than ever, because breast-feeding or not, you'll need extra energy to get your mojo back and look after baby.

If you're already well versed in keeping a green and clean kitchen, feel free to skip to the cool recipes. But if you're like I was, and the kitchen drawers look a lot like they did the day you moved in, read on. There are a bunch of things to learn: not only what to eat, but how to cook, store, and reheat, too. And in case you're worried the recipes are coming from me, the "order-in queen," fear not! For this chapter I have chosen two Green Gurus, each with her own method of feeding and eating. One is a green version of Rachael Ray, who keeps her pantry well stocked with heat-and-eat staples, such as organic canned green beans; the other is the green Martha, who would rather bake her own organic bread than have her kids chomp on store-bought. The strategies you choose are up to you. *Bon appétit!*

Green Guru

Karen Gurwitz

FOUNDER, MOTHERS & MENUS

AUTHOR, *THE WELL-ROUNDED PREGNANCY COOKBOOK*

MOTHER

Gurwitz was inspired to start Mothers & Menus, a natural-meal delivery service, when during her four-week-old's nap she had to choose between showering, eating, or resting. She thought, "How silly is it that I need to make that choice?" and looked for a business that could deliver the healthful meals she needed to take care of herself and her baby. When she couldn't find it anywhere, she started her own. Now fresh, delicious cooked meals can appear at new mothers' doors when they need them most. She also knows a lot about how to make cooking at home easier when you have a baby.

"What you really need to ask yourself is, 'What's the easiest way to create structure?' Don't plan on cooking every day.

When you do cook, make your meal work for you: Double ingredients and freeze leftovers for two or more meals. In my house, I cook for three hours on Sunday; then I have food for four days! I pull a meal from the freezer, reheat it, and add a leafy green.

"There are terrific organic broths available to speed up cook time and boost flavor. Get a package of each of your three favorite prepared veggies, baby carrots, frozen organic peas, whatever you love. Boil the broth, drop the veggies in, and simmer until tender. That's a hearty meal, or a satisfying starter packed with nutrients.

"Pregnancy gives you permission to take care of yourself in a way you don't otherwise do, and it's important to keep up the good work after baby is born, too. We are very good at meeting our deadlines and caring for others, but we have to remember to care for ourselves, as well. When you start looking at what you're doing every day, food is an easy way to do the right thing for yourself—I mean, you have to eat! Enjoy the difference organic makes."

Green Flag

You will likely only stick with plans that are easy, so you must find the easiest way to provide yourself and sometimes your mate with what you both need and enjoy.

- Keep on hand cans of organic beans and whole-grain rice.

- Prepacked, prewashed organic greens and veggies are a huge help.

• Fresh foods are better than canned, but using a mix of some canned and some fresh vegetables cuts prep time so much that I think it's worth it.

• Always opt for whole grains over super-processed.

• Shop around. I have found organic milk selling for anywhere from $2.99 to $4.99 a half gallon. And don't forget, you can check circulars and clip coupons for organic foods just as well as conventional.

• Buy smaller containers of organic ice cream, butter, and cheese. The flavor and richness are so superior, you might find you eat less. (This is good for your waistline, too!)

• When you find a good deal, like wild salmon on sale, buy a bunch and freeze it—ditto for pasture-raised chickens or free-range meat.

Green Guru

Jan Maltby
DOMESTIC DIVA
SUPER-GREEN MOM OF THREE

Jan is a full-time mom and volunteers at the Stone Barns Center for Food and Agriculture teaching children about the benefits of an organic farm. She has implemented an "edible classroom" with an organic greenhouse on the roof of her daughter's school and believes there are simple ways we can all integrate a healthy lifestyle into our daily routine.

"I often hear from people that they don't buy organic products because they're either too expensive or too hard to find. Organic products are more expensive because it costs more to pay farmers a fair living wage and to use more biodynamic methods to grow pesticide-free food. If you decide you want to adopt a greener lifestyle, here are a few ideas that might make it easier on your pocketbook and your life.

"Remember when bread machines were all the rage? Dust off the one that's in your cupboard or pick one up. You'll find them online or in most kitchen stores for about a hundred dollars. Finding fresh organic bread that stays fresh is tough. So every day, I take ten minutes to put all my organic ingredients into the machine, sit back, and wait for the aroma of baking bread to fill my house. My family loves the bread made with the recipe that follows. (You may have to adjust it for your machine.) Don't be afraid to experiment with pumpkin bread, cracked-wheat bread, or even brioche.

"My mother used to dry fruit leather on the picnic table in the summer. Since that is not very practical for me, I bought a food dryer. Again, this can be picked up online for about forty dollars. I use seasonal organic apples, apricots, tomatoes, bananas, strawberries, and just about anything else, stick it in my dryer, and forget about it for a few hours. You can also use your oven on a very low setting, but you will need to play with the temperature a bit. Either way, they are great treats for months to come at a fraction of the price at the store.

"Buy a cookbook that teaches you how to braise, the process of cooking slow and low in the oven with a small amount of herb-infused liquid. Cheaper cuts of meat are also ideal for this method. Crock-Pots cook a similar way, but braising creates a dish full of dense rich flavors. Each time you reheat your braised food, it just gets better.

"Go online and find an organic CSA in your neighborhood. 'CSA' is 'community-supported agriculture.' At the beginning of the season you invest in the farm. As each crop matures, you share its harvest. My CSA invites us to a farm picnic each year to complete the farm-to-table connection. The produce you receive will last far longer than anything you get from a conventional grocery, because you benefit from the lack of warehousing storage time and long-distance travel. Much of the time what I get from my CSA was literally picked earlier that day.

"Finally, go back to the Internet. Online stores like Amazon now offer bulk buying of nonperishable organic items. Watch for those free-shipping offers and go wild. Find a friend or two to share that case of unbleached chlorine-free paper towels, toilet paper, or nontoxic cleaning supplies if you don't have the space. You will be amazed how many nonperishable organic and healthy staples they offer and how much you will save."

Jan's Organic Honey Wheat Bread

3 tablespoons honey

2 tablespoons organic butter, softened

2 cups organic whole-wheat flour

1½ cups organic bread flour

1½ teaspoons salt

1¼ cups warm water

2 teaspoons yeast

Put all ingredients into the bread machine except water and yeast. Make 2 holes in the flour; fill 1 with the water and 1 with the yeast. Adjust the machine for a 1½-pound loaf, and turn it on.

Karen's Vegetarian Three-Bean Chili
SERVES 6 TO 8.

Don't let the long ingredient list fool you—preparing this dish is actually quick and easy; just keep in mind it needs to simmer for an hour. It can be stored in the refrigerator for 2 days, or in the freezer for up to 1 month. If you prefer some meat with your meal, add in 1 pound of browned grass-fed ground beef. Choose organic anything wherever you can.

3 tablespoons olive oil

1 can (15 ounces) black beans, rinsed and drained

1 medium sweet onion, chopped

1 can (15 ounces) red beans, rinsed and drained

1 medium carrot, chopped

2 jalapeños, seeded and minced

1 medium green, red, or yellow bell pepper, chopped (optional)

4 cloves garlic, minced

2 tablespoons chili powder

1½ teaspoons ground cumin

1 teaspoon ground coriander

1 teaspoon paprika

1 can (15 ounces) white beans, rinsed and drained

2 cans (16 ounces) plum tomatoes and their liquid, broken into chunks

1 sprig fresh thyme

1 bay leaf

½ teaspoon dried oregano

1 bottle (12 ounces) dark beer, preferably Mexican, or 1½ cups water

salt and freshly ground pepper

Heat the olive oil in a large heavy-bottomed saucepan over medium heat. Add the onion, carrot, jalapeños, and bell pepper; cook until the onion is translucent, about 5 minutes. Add the garlic, chili powder, cumin, coriander, and paprika; cook for 1 minute to bring out their flavors. The spices may stick to the pan—this is fine, just keep stirring.

Add the beans, tomatoes and their liquid, thyme, bay

leaf, oregano, and beer; bring to a boil. Cover, reduce the heat, and simmer for 1 hour.

Season with salt and pepper. Discard the thyme and bay leaf before serving.

Karen's Stir-fried Vegetables
with Curry Coconut Sauce
SERVES 2.

Beware: The following stir-fry is downright addictive. After you taste how its smooth, flavorful sauce contrasts perfectly with fresh, crunchy vegetables, you may never order take-out stir-fry again. Serve this delicious dish over rice, noodles, or quinoa. You can find curry paste at Asian markets or in health-food stores.

½ tablespoon canola oil

2 teaspoons peeled and grated fresh ginger

1 clove garlic, minced

4 ounces (1 cup) green beans, sliced on the bias into 1½-inch pieces

1 teaspoon sweet or hot curry paste

¾ cup canned coconut milk

salt and freshly ground black pepper

2 cups broccoli florets

1 medium carrot, peeled and cut into matchsticks

½ cup vegetable stock

2 tablespoons chopped scallions, white and light green parts only

2 tablespoons chopped toasted peanuts (optional)

½ cup cilantro leaves

In a large skillet, heat the oil over medium-high heat. Add ginger and garlic; cook for 1 minute. Add the green beans, broccoli, carrots, and stock; cover the pan and cook until the beans and florets have turned bright green, 1 to 2 minutes.

Stir the curry paste into the coconut milk. Increase the heat to high and add the curry mixture to the vegetables. Cook, stirring often, until the vegetables are crisp-tender, 3 to 4 minutes more. Add salt and pepper to taste. Stir in the scallions.

Sprinkle with chopped nuts and cilantro leaves before serving.

PLASTICS AND FOOD

Plastics are such a huge part of our lives—and our kitchens—that it might be tempting to just keep using them. What's not to like about plates that don't break when your fussy diva flings them to the ground? And plastic is probably at least part of her high chair, too. The containers for storing breast milk and freezing and reheating are, more often than not, plastic. Using plastic is so easy you might not feel motivated to look for an alternative. But before you turn a blind eye, there are several concerns you need to be aware of.

The following is a quote from "Get Plastic Out of Your Diet" by Paul Goettlich, director of www.mindfully.org. He has exhaustively researched how pervasive plastics are in, well, everything. He suggests we never allow plastics to come in contact with our food. While this is probably not possible for most of us, it's helpful to review his findings and consider his suggestions on limiting our use.

Bisphenol-A (BPA) is used in PC plastics, epoxy resins, and composites, and it is a heat stabilizer in PVC. The list of products containing BPA is long. Some rigid plastic containers, such as water and baby bottles, are made of PC plastics. The Consumer Union (CU) found BPA at worrisome levels in samples from baby bottles. CU advises its readers to avoid exposure to BPA by "dispos[ing] of polycarbonate baby bottles and replac[ing] them with bottles made of glass or polyethylene, an opaque, less-shiny plastic that does not leach bisphenol-A."

The Born Free company, in Austin, Texas, has started to manufacture baby products—including baby bottles and drinking cups—that do not contain phthalates or bisphenol-A. As reported in *Time* magazine in December 2006, Whole Foods Market stopped selling baby products that contain phthalates after reviewing "emerging scientific evidence of their risk."

WHAT'S YOUR NUMBER?

Plastic products and containers have numbers embossed on the bottoms. If you turn over a food container, you should be able to see a 1, 2, 3, 4, 5, 6, or 7, surrounded by a broken triangle. These numbers are codes that tell you what the plastic is made from. Items made of PVC and PS plastics have the numbers 3 and 6; these have the highest likelihood of leaching chemicals. Items made of polycarbonate have the number 7. Polycarbonate is a similar softer plastic, so you may want to avoid this one, as well.

Plastics with the numbers 1, 2, and 4 are made from polyethylene; those with the number 5 are made from polypropylene. These are widely considered safer alternatives.

If you do choose to use plastic containers, don't put them in the dishwasher or the microwave. Intense heat raises the possibility of chemicals leaching out. And don't be fooled by containers labeled "microwave safe"; this label only indicates that the item won't melt in the microwave, not that it is inherently "safe." For reheating, use containers made of glass or lead-free ceramic instead.

Red Flag

 Plastics 3, 6, and 7

Green Flag

 Plastics 1, 2, 4, and 5

When freezing food, let it cool down on its own before putting it into the freezer, so the hot food will not react with the container's surface. Again, plastic is more likely to leach into food under "stressful" conditions, such as heat. The safest alternatives for freezing are containers made from tempered glass or lead-free ceramic.

Use baby bottles free of bisphenol-A!

Barbara Haumann
THE ORGANIC TRADE ASSOCIATION

The Organic Trade Association was set up in 1985 to suggest, implement, and oversee guidelines for exactly what "organic" is. The OTA advocates and advances the organic message in Washington. The OTA serves all of North America from farm to home. In an (organic) nutshell, there would be no real criteria for organics, and in a sense no organics at all, without the OTA.

"I came to the Organic Trade Association in 1999. It's my job to speak and write about organics. People always say, 'Organic is not new—it's just going back to the way we used to do things.' But that's not true. In the old days, farmers farmed, then moved off the land. That's what the wagon trains were, farmers farming until the soil went dry, then moving on. That's not really sustainable. And that's not possible anymore, anyway. Organic is about learning to build the soil to be healthier. The first few years after a farmer converts to organic, his yields go down. Eventually he returns to his former level of production, and then the yields are higher, because he has restored the fertility of the soil. Organic farming produces agricultural products in a way that is healthy—for the land, the farmer and farm family, the local community, and the planet as a whole.

"Part of the tremendous growth of organic farming is the increased consumer demand; part of it is farmers rediscovering the joy of farming. Many smaller farmers converting to organic farming are saying, 'I love to farm, but I don't love to use pesticides.' Organic farming offers farmers the opportunity to live and thrive in a nice, healthy environment. We are seeing farmers' markets blossom, and big stores embrace particular family farmers. People want the connection to their food; they want to hear the stories, meet the farmers. I grew up on a farm where we raised our own food, and we weren't rich, but I never knew that. We ate so well. We ate well and we wanted to share that joy with others."

IN THE BAG

For some of us, the crinkly sound of cellophane just makes us salivate—we are so used to packaged and prepared foods. If you have succeeded in pretty much getting that munching monkey off your back for the sake of baby in the belly while you're pregnant, stick to your focus and try to continue to eat healthy and fresh whenever you can. However, sometimes, to keep our energy up, between our super-busy schedules and that extra little mouth to feed, it just makes sense to eat and run. So what do you choose? An organic apple or banana is a good idea, but if you need something a little more satisfying (and less prone to get mushy in the diaper bag), consider an energy bar.

THINK IT OVER Lizanne Falsetto makes the best munchies for folks on the go. A former model and now mother of two, Lizanne was looking for a better way to eat on the run, so she founded Think Products, the second-largest natural-energy-bar company in the country. "I know from experience that when you feel good, you can accomplish so much more," Lizanne says, "and what you put in your body directly affects how you feel. My Think Green bar contains only organic and natural ingredients and gives you what you need to keep keepin' on." Look for Lizanne's new Think 5 bars. One yummy bar has five full servings of fruits and veggies in a convenient package. I know this sounds impossible, but they are so addictive they've replaced my craving for Hershey's. (Later, this can be a kid's favorite, too!)

GREEN AT A GLANCE

Evergreen: Join community-supported agriculture. Get fresh fruits and veggies and be part of the solution. Check out localharvest.org for a CSA near you.

Pea green: Get organic staples at the supermarket and stock your cupboard. When you have the time, you can make the best meals yourself.

Spring green: Reconsider your food storage containers. Eschew those labeled 3, 6, and 7 in favor of those labeled 1, 2, 4, and 5.

Part III 🍃

Your
Green Baby:
Organically
Growing

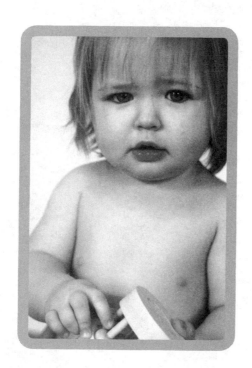

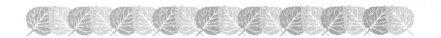

So you baby-proofed your home. Nice work! Unfortunately, you can't gate out the whole wide world.

It was hard enough inside the house, where you have to nail down everything from Grandpa's antique rocker to that cool mission floor lamp (what was that crash?)—how crazy do you have to go to keep your little tumble-bumble safe now that he's on the prowl? We'll look at some of the biggest concerns in your home now that baby is moving about like some Cirque du Soleil acrobat. Then, onward: Our new mission is to seek out new life and new civilization, to boldly go where your baby has not gone (much) before. Outside, the final frontier!

And yes, it does take a village to raise a baby. We'll tell you how to ensure your village is peaceful and toxin free, and how a love of the environment is related to a love of life and a love of self. We'll give you the tools to take on the surprisingly easy and fun task of inspiring greatness, and greenness, in those around you.

Finally, the answer we've all been waiting for: Who is going to protect baby from all these potential hazards, and at the same time make the world a better, more inviting place for all living things? Well, you'll just have to read the next chapter to find out. . . .

Eleven

How Green Was My Valley?

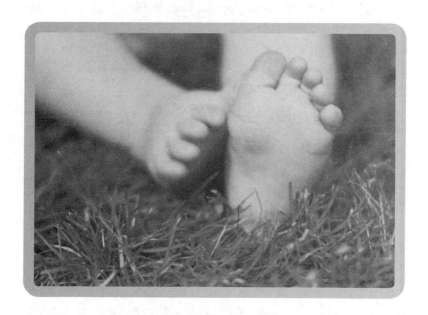

How to Keep Your Baby in the Pink While Playing on the Green

If you're lucky enough to have your own backyard, you will be using it—a lot—especially when baby is big enough to crawl around. If you don't have a backyard, you'll probably be headed for the town green or city park. Babies need the outside stimulation to grow and explore. But what's out there? What needs baby-proofing in the great outdoors?

Outside as well as in, baby explores things with his hands and mouth. So just like inside your home, outside the most important thing to do is to avoid pesticides. As you already know, pesticides are poison.

I know you're probably thinking, OK, I can control what goes on inside my house, but when we go out the front door, how can I control what other people do? And is it even my business? You bet it is. Pesticides do not follow property lines. They drift over fences and lawns, and they're brought into your backyard by squirrels and birds, giving new meaning to the song "This Land Is Your Land, This Land Is My Land." You can help your neighbors become good neighbors if you supply them with a few facts. It might sound uncomfortable. Actually, it is. It is uncomfortable to saunter next door, or across the street, ring the bell, and say you want to talk about their pest management. So before you do it, plan your course of action; pull together some facts and be specific about your concerns. Your neighbors are no different from you. They're perfectly nice people who just may be poisoning the plants, wildlife, and air on your street with the products they are using on their lawns. They don't *want* to harm you or your baby; they're just under the impression that what they are doing, and using, is safe. But if they're using a conventional pesticide or herbicide (the fancy name for weed killer), it probably isn't. By its very nature, something that is developed to kill is not safe. "Tolerable risk" is not even measured in terms of children's exposure. I had this problem with a kindly older couple who lived across the street from us. I remedied it with a spoonful of (organic) sugar. Here's what happened:

I used to go crazy when I'd see the little white poison truck pull up and dole out who knows what on my neighbors' lawn. Of course, the worker was always wearing a mask, but I wasn't. He'd come about once a month in the spring and summer. I wondered, "What do they have over there that they are so desperate to kill, Sasquatch?" When the little yellow WARNING! flags were stuck all over the lawn, I'd hurriedly close my windows. It made me so mad. Really mad. But I was friendly with them, and I knew a confrontation would be awkward, to say the least. So I cooked up a plan. And as I did so, I also cooked up some fabulous quiche— the one dish I am famous for is my organic spinach, garlic, and cheddar quiche. I covered it, crossed the street, knocked on the door, offered it up, and was invited in. We each had a slice of my savory pie. The compliments about my delish dish were rolling, and a recipe was asked for, giving me the opportunity to extol the virtues of organic agriculture, and the dangers of conventional farming and pest-management techniques. My neighbors told me that they had a terrible problem with wasps and were always spraying to get rid of them. I told them to be careful, that pesticide exposure is linked to many diseases, including Parkinson's. The next day I slipped some information on natural pest-management techniques under their door. I never saw the little white truck again. And we subsequently shared many more organic quiches together.

Green Guru

Jay Feldman
DIRECTOR, BEYOND PESTICIDES

Under the Carter administration, Jay spent several years in rural America working on the delivery of health-care services to farmworkers. He cataloged how workers were exposed to pesticides in the fields. The illnesses and the miscarriages he saw among those farmworkers prompted him to work to educate people about the hazards of pesticides. Note that many of the same chemicals that are used on farms are used on backyard lawns and public parks.

"The best way to avoid pesticides is to avoid pests. Organic landscaping is working very effectively to create and maintain beautiful lawns and yards.

"Some communities are going very clean and green. But some states are restricting local governments from more strictly regulating chemical lawn care. Villages and towns really need to see that chemical lawn care has a direct effect on the health and well-being of their communities. When you think about it, it's pretty reasonable. Secondhand pesticide exposure is just like secondhand smoke. And the use of weed killers and synthetic fertilizers creates a toxic runoff into waterways. The chemicals go directly into ecosystems and waterways, and the effects clearly are being felt. The chemical 2,4-D is regularly used in public parks and grasses bordering playgrounds, and it is being tracked indoors on your shoes. Half of Agent Orange, the infamous defoliant used in Vietnam, is composed of 2,4-D.

"We shouldn't have to be exposed to chemicals when we have access to safe and effective alternatives. There's a mindset that says, 'I need to buy conventional weed and feed products to have a good-looking lawn,' but that's just not true. We can use products that enhance a healthy environment or we can use products that do exactly the opposite.

"Earthworms naturally fertilize and aerate soil. Not every bug is a bad bug, but when you kill one, you can kill them all: the good and the bad ones.

"Children are most vulnerable in the years from birth through age five, when they are taking in the most air and water per pound of body weight and there is so much hand-to-mouth activity. We just can't continue to expose our kids to the serious, and invisible, risk that widespread pesticide use brings. We need to make this a priority in our communities.

"There have been some changes for the better: Marblehead, Massachusetts, has a policy that dictates public fields must be managed organically. Dane County, Wisconsin, has restricted the use of conventional weed and seed products. New York City just adopted a clean plan patterned after those in place in San Francisco and Seattle. Concerned people really need to call their local municipalities and make it known that this is an issue that is important to them."

You can't live inside all the time—and of course, you don't want to. It's a beautiful world, and baby needs to go out and about. So pick your battles and manage your risk:

• Ask yourself where you can have the greatest impact. Is it your own backyard? Can you organize a block party around natural lawn care where you share seeds and extra bulbs?

• Identify where your child spends most of her time. Make it a priority to be sure it is pesticide free.

• Call municipal offices to find out the lawn-care policies in your park district. If you are not happy with them, research alternatives and contact your elected officials with them.

You just never know what's been applied to the soccer field where you and baby watch your niece play, or to the backyard of your boss' home, where she holds her annual barbecue. Keep a big blanket in the car, or even a thin sheet rolled up in the diaper bag, for baby to crawl around on. Closely monitor any grass pulling and tasting. Wash the blanket or sheet in hot water and baking soda and vinegar before using it again.

NATURAL LAWN CARE

According to PlantTalk Colorado (www.ext.colostate.edu/ptlk), when a pest or disease is devastating your plants, refrain from grabbing the strongest chemical you can find. Always try simple, safe controls before using a pesticide:

• Sometimes a strong blast of water from a hose is all it takes to get rid of a pest.

• You can handpick pests like caterpillars and drop them into soapy water. (My kids, however, consider caterpillars a part of the family, so we'd remove them and drop them in a jar, then deposit them on a portion of the backyard that we had designated as the kids' garden. The kids had a butterfly bush as an anchor and had planted lots of hearty bloomers like sunflowers, milkweed, and even dandelions. We bordered it in mint, so they didn't go totally out of control. It was a haven for happy creepy-crawlers, kept my youngest from weeping, and ensured at least an occasional bloom in *my* corner of the yard.)

• Shake Japanese and potato beetles off plants onto a sheet. (If you're feeling vegan peace and love for the little critters, take them down to that vacant lot on the corner and shake 'em onto the wildflowers.)

• Aphids, cabbage worms, and white flies are attracted to the color yellow, so they can be trapped by covering a piece of yellow poster board with glue and hanging it among the infested plants.

• Ladybugs are actually not so ladylike at all: They are voracious carnivores and would love to pig out on your aphids. You can actually order a bagful from naturescontrol.com for about eight dollars. (My kids had a blast letting them go and we were aphid free and full of roses within a couple of weeks!)

• Dish-washing soap is a big turnoff for most insects, especially rose-chomping beetles. One part liquid dish soap to four parts water is generally mild enough for the plants but a persuasive deterrent for bugs.

• Vinegar is a great natural herbicide. Put equal parts vinegar and water in a spritzer bottle and zap even stubborn weeds.

• Google is a godsend. Before applying anything to your garden, identify the pest or disease you want to control so you can choose the most effective product.

PLEASE . . . COMPOST YOURSELF! The best fertilizers are also the cheapest. Prepare a compost pile in a shaggy corner: Just take biodegradable food trash and drop it in, and let the little wigglers do their stuff. Turn it over every week or two to aerate and in eight weeks, you've got gardeners' black gold! (Remember to use organic trash if you are planning on eating from your garden. There's no point in composting and recycling pesticides.)

A LITTLE TIGER IN ALL OF US
Golf courses are Godzillan guzzlers of water and also of pesticides.

Have you ever noticed that you never get bitten by a mosquito on the golf course, even when you're standing by the topiary? There are not many bugs that can survive the constant onslaught of chemicals used on most private courses.

If you can't—or don't want to—break the habit of goin' to the green, consider using your passion for the game to sway the club where you play into taking a more environmental approach.

A few lush golf courses and country clubs are now adopting more environmentally responsible practices.

In the meantime, be vigilant about where you put anything that was on you or with you while you were golfing, since it will absolutely carry an invisible but potent chemical coating when you leave.

And please think long and hard before taking a child onto a conventional golf course. Because they are small and their bodies are still growing and developing, toxins have a much greater effect on them.

HOP ON THE BUS, GUS

When we moved about ten years ago, our oldest daughter hadn't started school yet, but one of the reasons I fell in love with our house was that there was a school-bus stop on the corner. From a window in Layla's room I would see four or five buses come in the dark of early morning to pick up everyone from beaming kindergartners to lanky, sullen teens. And again I'd hear the rumble of the buses every afternoon when they brought the children back home.

Seeing them every day gave me a sense of comfort, like everything was going right in my little world. Things seemed as they should be and I delighted in imagining my child growing up and taking her seat on one of those yellow wonders.

But those buses are not the warm and fuzzy haven I thought they were. They leave a toxic trail of diesel exhaust along my street, and every street, exposing the kids who ride on them to the same. Worse yet, sometimes parents seeing young ones off to school have babies in tow—babies who, with every breath, are taking in toxic fumes as one idling bus after another waits for passengers.

John Wargo, professor of Risk Analysis and Environmental Policy at Yale University, has studied the risks associated with school-bus emissions. His work has been instrumental in enacting safer bus procedures, but procedures differ from state to state, and they can be very hard to enforce. He found that more than ninety-nine percent of U.S. school buses are powered by diesel fuel, yet most federal agencies call diesel exhaust a probable human carcinogen. There is no known safe level of exposure to diesel exhaust for children, especially those with respiratory illness.

According to Dr. Wargo, "If airways are inflamed or constricted by asthma, allergies, or infections, exposure to diesel exhaust may make breathing more difficult."

He goes on to suggest, "The current fleet of diesel-powered buses should soon be retrofitted with interior air filters, particle traps, and catalytic converters capable of trapping ultrafine particles, and be powered by ultralow-sulfur fuels."

Red Flag

Unless or until you can avoid the bus fumes altogether, do not stand downwind of a waiting bus, and instruct your child and other children to follow suit.

Don't bring siblings to the bus stop if you can leave them at home with another adult.

Green Flag

Ask your school transportation department what their policy is on idling buses in the afternoon load-on periods, when children are most likely to be exposed to the most buses and their exhaust. Insist ignitions are turned off as kids get on and wait to leave.

Talk about this in your community. Push for tougher regulations on idling time, and ask for more filters on school buses.

ARSENIC AND OLD PLACE: *TOXIC PLAYGROUNDS AND OTHER REMNANTS OF OUR CHEMICAL PAST*

Wooden park benches and playground equipment—like cotton, they sound so natural, and are such a given, accepted part of our lives, that we all assume they must be safe and OK. But just as with conventional cotton, they contain hidden dangers you probably didn't know about.

Most of the pressure-treated "outdoor" wood used to make playground equipment, decks, and picnic tables is preserved with the arsenic-containing chromated copper arsenate, or CCA. The EPA began its phaseout of sales of arsenic-treated wood for residential uses in December 2003. But there were few stipulations for existing private structures. So decks, outdoor furniture, and wooden playground sets that were built or purchased before December of 2003 are probably laced with arsenic. Public benches and playground equipment vary wildly from community to community. Some have recently been replaced with aluminum or plastic, others sealed to reduce transferring the toxins. Sealing is only a temporary measure at best, and one that must be done a few times a year to be effective. The bench you're sitting on by the playground may well be leaching arsenic onto your exposed skin. Arsenic, even in very small amounts, is known to cause skin, lung, and bladder cancer, and is linked to diabetes, heart disease, and other health problems. Children have the highest risk for two reasons: They are the ones most likely to be spending the most time in parks and on playground equipment, and their smaller, still-developing bodies are more vulnerable to toxins. Some studies estimate that one in five hundred children who regularly play on arsenic-treated wood playgrounds may develop fatal cancer later in life due to this exposure.

You'll never be able to avoid all arsenic-treated wood because it's all around us. It was used to build docks on piers, telephone poles, school playground equipment, and many park benches. Exposure to even very low levels of arsenic is hazardous because part of it is chromium 6, the chemical made famous by Erin Brockovich. So it's important to remove as much of it as you can from your child's life.

If you have a deck around your house, or a wooden play set you didn't install yourself, and you're not sure of the year it was manufactured, be sure to have the wood tested. Tests cost around a hundred dollars. Your local municipal authority will help you find someone to conduct these tests. You'll need to take a scraping, send it away, and wait for the lab results.

GETTING FRIENDS AND RELATIVES TO GO FOR THE GREEN

Sure, your whole life has totally changed, but that doesn't necessarily mean that everyone else's has. (What!? Not changing their whole lives for your baby? Humph . . . I pity the fools!)

Sometimes, even loving friends and family can get miffed if they feel like they're being pushed too hard to join your green team.

I clearly remember when my mother-lioness instinct first showed itself—and the disappointing result. We were living in downtown Manhattan, on Second Avenue and Twelfth Street. Our neighborhood, the East Village, was known as a haven of both urban chic and decay, and with good reason. When I was struck with an urge to shop, Eileen Fisher's first store was just two blocks away and I was surrounded by countless other tiny milliners and designers who were often featured in *Vogue* and other stylish glossies. But across the street from our apartment was the St. Mark's churchyard, to which I trudged many a frigid night to drop off blankets to the homeless who had parked on the benches for the night. (My DAR grandmother had for many years saved those fine wool blankets in a cedar chest for my children. Sometimes I would later see them swathing neighborhood transvestites in full Diana Ross coiffure and eye makeup. Gramma would not have approved.)

Anyway, it was a wonderful time for me and my little family. Our neighborhood was colorful, but the streets were not exactly Switzerland clean, if you get what I mean. So when a cousin of my husband's, a well-known jazz musician who lived farther east in the Village than we did, dropped by to see little four-week-old Layla, I asked him to leave his shoes at the door and please stop in the bathroom and wash his hands. He tilted his head, looked me in the eye, and said, "My hands are clean. I washed them before I left my house." Well, on his way over he had touched who knows what. He most definitely touched the downstairs doorbell, the outside door, the inside door, and the elevator buttons. He was bringing in, basically, the whole bloomin' neighborhood! We got into an argument, and even though he finally did remove his shoes and wash his hands, it was not the warm and fuzzy family gathering I had hoped for. Looking back, I could have handled this situation differently, and perhaps gotten everything I wanted instead of the argument and resulting migraine that followed.

Here are a couple of ways to make the baby transition easier on friends and relatives:

• Consider making a little sign near the door that says SHOES. You can always greet your guests with a kiss on the cheek and glance at the sign and say (sweetly), "Do you mind?"

• Instead of immediately passing your anxiety on to your visitors, hug them and say, "Oh, I can't wait for you to meet baby! Can I show you where you can wash up? We are trying to keep fragrances to a minimum so I have a special soap. . . ." They may think you've lost it, but who could say no after a hug?

With a little love and a lotta charm you can be like fantastic Frank Sinatra—"I did it my way"—and get what you want. But sometimes, especially if you're not on your own turf, it won't be so easy to do as you please. When people's actions conflict with the parenting style you're trying to practice, take stock of the situation and ask yourself:

• What's the downside if things don't go your way? Is baby potentially in danger?

• Instead of fight or flight, can you add one more possible reaction: *flow*? Is this something you can just let go or will it cause enough concern to spoil the encounter?

• Do you have a good reason and can you convey it rationally and nonjudgmentally?

• Does Mother know best right now? Try to just breathe. It is possible that you may be a little crazed from your hormones and ferocious love. Your friends and family members want the best for your baby. They love you—that's why they're in your life. So when their actions aren't *really* putting your baby at risk, it's better, sometimes, to take a deep breath and follow the advice of lyricist Steve Winwood: "Roll with it, baby!"

If, on the other hand, you are pretty sure your concerns have merit, stand up for yourself, and do what you feel is right. Your mother instincts are a powerful asset to your parenting work, so listen up; baby is counting on you.

Red Flag

Don't demand people make sweeping, onerous changes.
Don't demand they do everything exactly as you do.
Don't demand, period! Ask graciously.
Don't criticize or psychoanalyze their woeful blunders.

Green Flag

Make your requests specific and limited in scope.
Explain your reasons. Be prepared with facts. If nothing else, it can be helpful to depersonalize by saying, "My pediatrician says . . ." rather than, "I feel . . ."
Assume everyone means well, unless proven otherwise.

GREEN AT A GLANCE

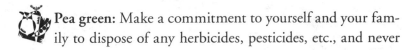 **Evergreen:** Become a voice in your community. Stampede your local municipal building and demand that the people there protect your children. (OK, OK. Don't literally stampede. But do make yourself heard. You know, save the playground, save the world!)

Pea green: Make a commitment to yourself and your family to dispose of any herbicides, pesticides, etc., and never buy or use chemical lawn care again. Call your local municipality to find out hazardous-waste days for garbage pickup. In the meantime, store them out of the way of wandering little ones.

Spring green: Have your deck and outdoor wooden furniture tested for arsenic. Take steps to seal or remove if you get bad news. (Keep in mind arsenic is so toxic that the soil surrounding the structure will be contaminated, as well.)

Twelve

Give Peas a Chance

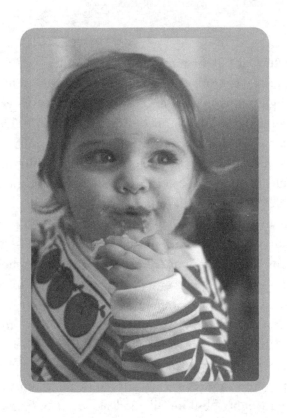

When the Outside World
Enters Your Baby's Mouth

We started our first baby on solids under very weird and stressful circumstances. Like many milestones in my journey through motherhood, the experience was very different from what I had imagined, or planned. It was the winter of Layla's first year, and we were still living in our apartment in Manhattan. The news was filled with reports of a huge impending snowstorm that would blanket the Northeast. What that meant for most (smart) New Yorkers was a quick trip to the neighborhood grocery store or corner bodega to stock up on staples like milk and bread. But what a blizzard meant to my husband—who had spent many of his vacations from British boarding school in the Swiss Alps—was an opportunity, a siren call, really, to go skiing. So he rented an SUV (we were unaware of global warming then), and we headed off to Stowe, Vermont, with our five-month-old in tow. Well, the trip up was downright terrible. There was zero visibility. A huge portion of the other silly people who had ventured out were stranded in their cars to our left and right, with their hazard lights blinking like sad old neon bar signs. About two hours into the trip, which would take at least five hours on a good day, Layla started crying. Howling, really. We pulled over and I took her out of her car seat to nurse her. I had exclusively

breast-fed her since birth, and she had never had any other sustenance of any kind. (And she ate all the time! That's how I got rid
of my extra baby weight. You cannot possibly eat enough to keep
extra pounds on if your baby exclusively breast-feeds, believe me.
I used to chow down at least a quart of Häagen-Dazs every night,
and I still effortlessly shrank back to a size six!)

OK, I'll wrap up the story of the Long Day's Journey into Food.
Layla continued to scream and cry.

We stopped at a little gas station/mini-mart with my shrieking
bundle. The kindly old lady at checkout told me she thought the
baby was hungry and suggested we get some Gerber cereal; for
some reason, even though I thought she was daft, I bought the
cereal! We continued our journey, with me now sitting in the back
attempting to console, distract, and shut up my baby in a nice,
motherly way. When nothing else was working, I mixed the cereal
with some bottled water and spoon-fed it to her. She ate it all,
smiled, gurgled, and zonked out.

So that was the beginning of my baby becoming her own
person —and also the beginning of the stinky poops. (No one had
told me that my baby's sweet-smelling doodie, which didn't smell
at all when she was only on breast milk, would immediately become stink bombs as soon as she started eating solid foods!)

But those weren't the only sad parts. Because my baby was eating "something else," her insides were exposed to the whole wide
world of agriculture and technology. I realized I now had to be
especially vigilant about knowing what was passing by her sweet
little lips, and where it came from, because that was the "stuff"
that would grow my baby.

We never fed her conventional baby food again. Thank goodness
the people of Vermont were forward-thinking enough, even back
then, to have Earth's Best, the first certified-organic baby food.

I've since had two more babies and many, many years of feeding children (in fact, I still am). Let's look at some of the reasons why organic food is the best choice for babies and kids:

- Pesticide use has increased thirty-three-fold in the United States since the end of the Second World War.

- Children eat, drink, and breathe more pesticides, pound per pound, than adults; plus their bodies are growing and developing.

- A study of Seattle schoolchildren showed that those who were fed nonorganic diets had six times the amount of pesticides in their urine than children who were fed organic diets.

- Recent studies have even linked behavioral difficulties with some food additives.

- In an editorial in the *Chicago Tribune*, Professor Robert Hatherill of the University of California, Santa Barbara, wrote, "A rapidly expanding body of research shows that heavy metals, such as lead and pesticides, decrease mental ability and increase aggressiveness. Rather than directing all of our attention to bitter debates on gun control and the violence in the entertainment industry, let's also consider the pressing need for a cleaner environment."

- According to the National Children's Study, which was mandated by Congress in 2000, ADHD and developmental disorders collectively are estimated to affect eighteen percent of all schoolchildren—nearly one in every five. Childhood-cancer rates jumped twenty-one percent from 1975 to 1998 and continue to rise about one percent each year. Cancer is now the leading disease that kills children under age fifteen in the United States.

• According to Charles Benbrook, the chief scientist at the Organic Center (www.organic-center.org), "New information from the USDA's Pesticide Data Program shows that from 2004 to 2005, there was a significant increase in residues of synthetic pyrethroids in milk. Today, about forty-five percent of conventional milk samples contain a residue of a pyrethroid insecticide."

Pesticide exposure poses a very significant risk to the development of babies and children. Any conventional (nonorganic) food your child eats raises his pesticide exposure in two ways: First, there are the pesticides he is ingesting with the food. Second, when you buy nonorganic foods, you are supporting agribusinesses that pollute the soil and groundwater. There just isn't a magic garbage barge that takes these poisons off the planet. We are at a critical point in determining the health of children in the United States. It's time we cleaned up our act, and one of the easiest and most certain ways to do it is to choose organic products. Consider it a deposit in your green bank. As others do the same, our combined resources create a healthy playing field for all our children to grow and flourish on.

For lots of great information, check out the industry-leading nonprofit organization the Organic Center (www.organic-center. org), which researches the scientific reasons organic is better, and shares its research with the world.

I've got Green Gurus galore for you in this chapter, because one thing is for sure: Your baby will be eating food every day for the rest of his life! And I want to share with you the best info from the smartest green foodies in the baby biz, so you can make the most informed decisions about the building blocks of your baby's body.

Green Guru

Kim Bremer
BRAND MANAGER, EARTH'S BEST BABY FOOD
MOTHER OF TWO

Earth's Best is the industry leader in a market that is exploding: organic baby food. Earth's Best is all-organic. If, like me, you don't have the time, energy, or inclination to peel, steam, and freeze food yourself, you can use Earth's Best as a trusted, easy, and convenient way to protect your baby from pesticides. And you won't be alone. Green armies of new moms are loading it into their shopping carts.

"I'm a mother of two young children, and I'm expecting my third. I also have a full-time job. So while I want the foods my kids eat to be healthy and nutritious, I also need them to be convenient. It's important to be able to get what your child wants to eat in the place you shop. Fortunately, chances are you can find lots of organic choices, including Earth's Best, right in your area.

"Earth's Best is twenty years old. It was started in Vermont by two brothers who looked at jarred baby food and wondered why it had so many additives, fillers, and sugars. They wanted to make something very pure, very natural, and today we're not just the oldest jarred-organic-baby-food company but the largest and strongest, as well. We have more than seventy-five varieties of jarred foods, organic whole grains, even soups.

"Even when your kids aren't babies anymore, you can feel good about giving them things like organic applesauce for their lunch box or whole-grain pasta for dinner. Crunchin' Cheddar Crackers imprinted with Elmo and Big Bird make my own little ones chuckle!

"Believe me, I know that organic needs to be delicious, accessible, and easy in order to be part of your daily life."

Green Guru

Shazi Visram
FOUNDER, HAPPY BABY FROZEN GOURMET BABY FOOD

There's a terrific new option that wasn't available when mine were little tykes: organic frozen baby food. It's a great middle ground between traditional jars and cooking from scratch. (Plus it offers a bridge between our healthy, affluent kids and children who don't have as much. For every box purchased, Happy Baby feeds an undernourished child in Malawi for a day.)

"I had the idea to do something fresh for baby way back in 2003. I was in business school at Columbia and a dear friend had just had twins. She's an amazing woman, a kind of icon, someone who does everything wonderfully. But one day she confided how bad she felt about how she was feeding her kids. She had imagined making every meal for them herself, especially their first bites. But when it came down to it, she felt a little overwhelmed. I thought, for baby's first foods, there's got to be something better—and I'm gonna do it!

"The first couple of years are about developing taste. If the first tastes you have are of super-processed or sugary foods, this is what you later associate with sustenance and comfort. First foods are first food experiences—and you are bound to repeat them. Our friend and supporter Dr. Bob Sears says moms should have their babies try a lot of fruits and veggies, because it makes for less picky eating later. And no one wants a picky toddler!

"We want to deliver the absolute best product. That means all our products are certified organic. We fast-freeze our food, because that's the best way to preserve nutrients. And it's in convenient, one-cube-at-a-time, ready-to-reheat servings. So you can pop out and reheat what you need, and put the rest back in the freezer to reduce waste."

Green Guru

Joan Ahlers and Cheryl Tallman
OWNERS, FRESH BABY SO EASY BABY FOOD KITS
AUTHORS, *SO EASY BABY FOOD*
MOTHERS

The Fresh Baby So Easy Baby Food Kit makes doing the right thing pretty foolproof (and this is coming from me, the modern-day *I Love Lucy*!). It comes with a baby-food cookbook that explains everything; two (food-safe) freezer storage trays, which are like ice-cube trays with a nifty cover on them that makes them spill-proof and stackable in the freezer (the trays are made out of a PVC-free high-density plastic that doesn't leach and contains no bisphenol-A or plasticizers); and a how-to DVD. These two are the real deal. They are both true-blue green entrepreneurs. Joanie already had four children when, from across the country, her sister Cheryl asked for advice and help with her first. Here's their story.

"Our mom was a natural mom. We were all breast-fed and she always encouraged us to eat healthy foods," Joan says. "I remember when I started my first baby on solid food. I bought a few jars of baby food at the store, came home, and opened a jar of peas, only to find that it just didn't smell or look like peas—I assumed it was bad. I tossed it and opened another only to discover the same thing. I picked up the phone and called Mom for advice. She told me it would be easy to make my own baby food—just steam and puree fresh produce. This simple suggestion sent me on my path to make baby food for all four of my children and I got better at it with each one."

"Joanie had a whole system for making baby food," Cheryl says. "But I was like, 'No way, I do *not* have time.' But she gave me a five-minute pitch on how healthy fresh food was, how easy it was to make baby food, and that it took less than thirty minutes a week. So I trusted my little sister and I was so surprised—she was right! I came from a marketing background and thought, 'Why don't we package something so other people can do this, too?' People do know that fresh is best—they just might not know how to do it or how little time it takes. Plus when I saw other parents with kids who struggled with weight problems, I noticed that they did not make their own food, but rather fed them processed foods. Our pediatrician agreed with me that fresh was best, and that if I kept it up, my kid would be much better off. He was right on the money—and speaking of money, it was a lot cheaper to make our own food, as well.

"Together Joanie and I started Fresh Baby so that all parents can have the option to make their baby food and enjoy all the benefits without having to reinvent the system for doing it."

Tips from Joanie and Cheryl

TEN HEALTHY EATING HABITS

1. Teach your baby about different fruits and vegetables.

2. Talk about what your baby is eating. Make it fun.

3. Be a role model. Your baby learns by mimicking you.

4. Encourage drinking water. Offer it at each meal.

5. Don't give up. Your baby's tastes will change daily.

6. Your baby needs a balanced diet. Offer plenty of variety.

7. Don't be in a rush at mealtimes. Relax and enjoy the time.

8. Set times for breakfast, lunch, snacks, and dinner.

9. Never force your baby to eat.

10. Make mealtime a family event. Avoid distractions.

FRESH-BABY-FOOD TIPS

• Keep your hands and all utensils clean while making and serving baby food.

• To prepare: Wash, peel, and cut, then stove-top steam or microwave in less than ten minutes. Create a smooth texture with a blender or food processor. (There's no such thing as overpureeing!) Pour into food trays and cover. Freeze overnight. Pop cubes out and store in freezer in an airtight container or a zip freezer bag. They'll last up to two months.

• To serve: Select frozen food cubes from freezer, place in dish, and thaw or warm. Stir food before serving. If you want to thicken something, use vitamin-fortified baby cereal, yogurt, or mashed banana. For thinning, use breast milk/formula, one hundred percent juice, or low-sodium soup stock.

• *Always* check the temperature of food before serving.

• You can mix different cubes together to create tasty meals. Try peas and sweet potatoes; green beans and white potatoes; broccoli, cauliflower, and melted cheese; butternut squash, corn, and tofu; peaches, pears, rice cereal, and ground almonds; or raspberries, apples, yogurt, and ground walnuts.

COMMON BABY AILMENTS AND FOODS

Ailment	Foods to Consider Avoiding	Foods That May Help
Diarrhea	High-fat foods	Bananas, rice, applesauce, toast, plain potatoes, plain pasta, clear liquids (water or broth)
Upset stomach, colic	Fried foods, citrus fruits, eggs, broccoli, cauliflower, garlic, onions, wheat	Potatoes, avocados, bananas, squash, raisins, ginger, rice, nuts, chamomile or peppermint tea (no caffeine)
Constipation		Water and fruit juice, prunes or prune juice, raisins, nuts
Runny nose	Dairy products	Increased fluids, apricots, broccoli, cauliflower, citrus fruits, kiwi, mango, papaya, strawberries, tomatoes
Teething pain		Frozen veggie sticks (cooked), wet washcloth to teethe on

Diaper rash	Broccoli, cauliflower, citrus fruits, kiwi, papaya, straw- berries, tomatoes	Yogurt with active cultures
Poor sleeping		Potatoes, bread, warm milk, pasta, turkey

Green Guru

Tricia McKelwee

GREEN BABIES ADVISER

CERTIFIED HERBALIST AND NUTRITIONIST

SUPER-GREEN MOM

Tricia always makes her baby's food. Here's how:

"I always enjoyed making my own baby food, but when babies start feeding themselves the chunky foods and they no longer primarily eat creamy, pureed foods, you can get more creative. This starts at about ten months.

"My focus is to make sure that at every meal she gets whole grains, legumes, and veggies along with added healthy fats (DHA, hemp, or flax oils).

"I am currently a stay-at-home mom but find that I am still very busy and simply don't have the time to prepare homemade meals all the time, so the food needs to be prepared whenever I can. On a morning or afternoon where I have a little bit of time, even if it's a half hour every now and then, I will make the following foods . . . and not all at once, just as we run low:

• Whole grains—brown rice, millet, and quinoa

• Legumes—I buy the beans and soak overnight . . . lentils, lima beans, pinto beans, chickpeas, etc.

• Veggies—broccoli, peas, carrots, cauliflower, zucchini

• Root veggies—sweet potatoes, squash

"I simply cook the foods, place in ice-cube trays (like you do when you make the pureed foods), and freeze overnight. When it's time for lunch or dinner, I grab a cube or two of whole grains and legumes, a handful of frozen veggies or some cubed squash or sweet potatoes. I warm the food in a steamer for twelve minutes. I went out and purchased one for probably thirty dollars. We do not use the microwave. The steamer ensures the most nutrients remain in her food.

"I drizzle the flax, hemp, or DHA oil onto her grains, slice up some fresh fruits, and voilà: in all of twelve minutes she has a healthy lunch of (for example) quinoa, broccoli, pinto beans, squash, and some strawberries. She gobbled this food down from ten months, no questions asked. Friends and family couldn't believe how healthy she ate and it was all nearly homemade in a few minutes.

"The keys are to buy organic, make ahead of time from each food group, freeze in cubes, reheat in steamer."

Whichever baby food you choose, I hope you'll explore treating yourself right, too.

My friend Annika Paradise tells this amazing story about awakening to the true nature of synthetic sweeteners: "When I was a Peace Corps volunteer in Thailand, I had a heck of a time keeping the ants away from food. I tried Raid, I even put the table legs into bowls full of water so my food had a moat. One day, a packet of Equal spilled onto the floor, and I watched these audacious ants that just walked over the Raid actually back away from the Equal. So then I started using Equal to keep the ants away from my food. I haven't put any artificial sweetener into my body from that day on."

If artificial sweeteners were not good enough for you (and baby) when you were pregnant or breast-feeding, they're really not good enough for you or the rest of your family at any other time, either. Most FD&C colors add to your body's chemical burden, too. Ever wonder what makes those cheese puffs such a brilliant orange? And do the words "toaster" and "strudel" really belong together? Good, fresh food doesn't hide behind artificial dyes and synthetic flavors. No matter how cute the name or tempting the ads, it's time to retrain our minds and our mouths to do the right thing for ourselves. We are so worth it, and our families are depending on us.

And as if it wasn't enough to check the ingredients in packaged foods, you also have to worry about the ingredients in the package itself. Beware of foods that come in packages treated with BHT. I've found it lurking in boxes of wholesome-looking things like oatmeal bars. BHT is a highly toxic chemical that is impregnated into the packaging to discourage rodents from nibbling through the box when foods are warehoused for long periods. So, assuming you don't have a household of Willard and friends, you probably don't want or need it in your kitchen cupboard.

Reading every word on every package can be a drag, but unless you frequent one of the super naturals—they don't stock products made with MSG or a host of other synthetic additives—it's worth your time to become an ingredient checker. Remember, it's just not possible to separate what we put *in* our bodies from what happens *to* our bodies. And you will want to be around for that impressive valedictorian speech baby will give one day!

KEEP THE HUMMER, BAN THE BURGERS!

(Oh, forget that—don't keep the Hummer, you gas hog!)

But here's some news: Trading in your Partridge Family–size SUV for a tiny hybrid is important, but not the number-one way you can do your bit for the planet. According to a University of Chicago study, becoming a vegetarian is actually a better way of combating global warming than swapping to a hybrid car. (There's nothing to prevent you from doing both, though!)

At the very least, consider giving up beef. Cows need space to chow down, space that could otherwise be used to grow crops to feed people. Energywise, you can have twenty veggie burgers for the energy price of one beef hamburger, but that's not all. . . .

Animals emit greenhouse gases. How? By farting. Yup, "he who smelt it, dealt it." So those cows are doing a whole lotta smelting (I mean "smelling"!). *Excusez-moi*, but did you know gaseous farm animals are responsible for about twelve percent of global methane?

So go veggie as much as you possibly can, and be kind to your four-legged friends, your heart, and your home: Earth.

All we are saying is give peas a chance.

GREEN AT A GLANCE

Evergreen: Opt to go veggie and replace animal-based proteins with plant-based combos.

Pea green: Choose organic whenever possible for grains, fresh fruits, and veggies as the basis of most meals for you and your family.

Spring green: Avoid synthetic flavors and colors in packaged foods.

Thirteen

Where Do Green Babies Come From?

Why, Sage Moms, of Course!

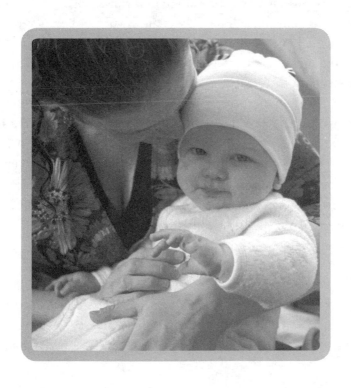

How to Make the Best
Choices for Your Child
and the Environment

For years my husband and I struggled with juggling our duties as parents and our responsibilities as business owners. I understand why entrepreneurs who break new ground are called "pioneers." It must have been tough on those wagon trains—an exhausting journey, followed by endless work to be done on arrival. It might not have been quite that brutal for us, but on many days and nights, it sure seemed like it. I remember taking naps on a jute rug on the cement floor of our warehouse between filling orders when I was expecting our youngest.

I used to haul my kids up the street to the converted fire station we used as a warehouse and have them do their homework on the cutting-room table while I scurried about to pack orders in time for the UPS pickup. My husband was schlepping back and forth from the factory in Queens to keep an eye on production and be sure our quality was top-notch. We worked so hard and such long hours, it's surprising we were even together enough to have so many kids.

People in the beautiful, bucolic town where we lived didn't seem to "get" us. I felt like an outsider, plowin' the land and building the ol' log cabin. From my perspective, my lucky neighbors seemed to have everything worked out.

Now I know that everybody else was really just like us: trying to keep it all together and love and care for their kids, while navigating the murky, uncharted territory called parenthood.

And looking back, I also think people just had no idea what we actually did. Absolutely nobody seemed to know what organic cotton was. Folks would innocently ask my husband, "Green Babies . . . what's that?"

And with a straight face, he'd say, "It's an adoption agency for Martian children." (Hmm, perhaps that explains those weird looks I got at the PTA meetings. . . .)

But seemingly overnight, everything changed. When our youngest daughter, Nadia, turned five and started going to school, it opened up a lot of possibilities for our time and our business. I remember, the evening of her birthday, telling my husband, "OK, now we should grow the business." The very next day, we got a call from Whole Foods Market. They are the world's largest, most credible and innovative natural-foods store. They told us they wanted to try a new concept, a baby boutique in their soon-to-be-built flagship store in Austin, Texas.

We told them we weren't sure how it would work. After all, we make baby clothes, and their middle name is, well, "Foods." But from the very beginning, Green Babies in Whole Foods Market was a big success. On the opening day, crowds waited outside and ran into the store, ecstatic with green goodness, grabbing our rompers off the shelves. It looked like a car-dealership commercial from the 1980s. It was a green dream come true.

We'd already enjoyed tremendous success. Our clothing had been on the covers of many magazines and seen on the babies of celebrities. But never before had we experienced the full force of this new, more-natural trend so up-close and personal. We came to understand that the overall driving force behind the growth of organics, fair trade, and conscious consumerism could be summed up in one powerful word:

Mothers.

We are it. We are the doorway to the future, the loving embrace, the decisive diplomat, and the bodyguard at the star's dressing-room door.

And why not? Our babies are the most important people in the world (as every baby is). Ambassadors from the future, they deserve diplomatic immunity and special treatment. And we are the prized personal assistant, the revered authority, the brilliant artist from which came this fab creation, this beautiful baby. We, mothers, are all that. . . .

It's no coincidence that necessity is the *mother* of invention. Mothers are inventing a whole new world.

For the first time ever in the history of humanity, we have, en masse, the freedom, the education, and the financial resources to reshape whatever we deem unfit in our children's world.

And a world that's truly safe for your child and my child is a shining, green, bountiful, and beautiful world for children everywhere.

OK, so what are the changes you need to make? What are the hurdles you need to overcome in order to excel at this most wonderful and rewarding of jobs?

Well, obviously, you need your sanity, your baby's health, and frankly, you need to take the reins and make sure, in the nicest way possible, that everyone knows who the boss is: you!

YOUR PIECE/PEACE OF MIND

Being a mom is a wonderful thing—but it can be very isolating and occasionally even downright lonely. Sometimes working moms feel reluctant to talk with coworkers or childless friends about the feelings and changes that motherhood brings. In the competitive climate of the workplace we don't want to be branded as a mushy mommy, someone who can't wait to leave work and run home to baby (even if it's true sometimes). And we certainly don't want to be insensitive to friends, who may already be feeling like we don't have much time for them anymore, by extolling the virtues of our new favorite person.

And the grass isn't necessarily greener on other side of the fence: Being a full-time mom can be equally lonely. Putting, basically, all our needs on hold to be at the constant beck and call of baby can be mind-numbing at times, and leaves many of us without a strong sense of self, even if we're embracing the bigger picture and really enjoying our new role as mom and primary caregiver.

Either way, I have one big fat piece of advice for you: *Do not go it alone!* Put yourself out there and connect with other like-minded mums.

IT TAKES A VIRTUAL VILLAGE

Welcome. You've got a lifetime membership to one big, happy club. Everyone on the planet has some connection to the birthin' thing and the experience of babyness (that's how we got here!). Yours is absolutely unique, but at the same time universal. It's wonderful, but things have changed. In fact, your whole day-to-day life as you know it has totally changed. That little welcome one is not like your dog (who lets you sleep at night, and allows you to go out to dinner occasionally, and have a shower before five p.m.). Baby needs to be fed, not once or twice, but all through the day! And baby can't do even the simplest things for himself. . . . Ugh! Can't you make it to the bathroom!? Oh yeah, I guess you can't. . . . But baby is amazing—just look at those eyelashes! Oh my gosh—did she just say "dada"? Baby is absolutely wonderful—truth be told, the most wonderful person ever to land on the planet. As cartoonist Don Herold said, "Babies are such a nice way to start people." And they certainly are. Unprepared as you may be, you are now in charge (of that little charge). You are Simon on *American Idol*, proclaiming what is actually good or bad, the way to go, or the wrong choice of a song. The future of the world was delivered from your loins and rests on your shoulders. . . . Seems like a pretty big responsibility to handle, just you and your mate. But don't worry, you're not alone; others are out there with you. And like you, they have a passionate and vested interest in getting this done right. You can do it, and the Internet is there at any hour of the day and night to help.

"In our crazy, busy days it's important to take a moment and just breathe," says Debra Flashenberg, who runs Manhattan's Prenatal Yoga Center. "Connecting to our breath is a way to remind you how strong you are. We're called Prenatal, of course, but we offer a lot of programs for new moms, too. Lots of women don't have their families around anymore, and there's a bond that happens to moms who meet in a prenatal class. I really suggest you try to keep in contact with those moms. You are going through a similar experience at the same time—you share a vast common ground. Now, because of the Internet, there is a huge community right at your fingertips!

"We started an online community in August 2006 with such a simple idea. We wanted to be of service to expectant and new moms. I'm a certified doula and have assisted at more than fifty births, so I have an idea of the kind of support women are looking for. If you're not near a lactation consultant and you have a question about breast-feeding, it's not a problem—we can connect you. There's a whole group of people out there who don't care if you're still in your jammies at five p.m. And it's important to have support. If your back is really killing you, we'll show you stretches. We'll give you two or three minutes of free yoga postures that should bring you relief! You're not alone. You should feel good about your experience!"

KEEPIN' IT GREEN

It can be hard to stick to your ideas and ideals when the real world enters. There's an old saying, "Anyone can keep a vow of silence if there's no one around to talk to." And this might as easily be said about keeping a green focus if you have the luxuries of time and sleep and all you have to worry about is you. But baby shrinks time and budgets, and sometimes inadvertently even strains family ties. Everyone's an "expert" and seems to have an opinion on what is the right way to feed, clothe, and generally do anything in regard to baby. But you, Mom, can stay true to your vision, and strengthen your information pool and resolve by gathering ideas and connecting with like-minded people online.

Following are some of the greenest online resources for information:

Green Guru

Jen Boulden
FOUNDER, IDEAL BITE

People with the superhuman patience of, say, a pointillist painter or kindergarten teacher have been known to measure the length of their shrunken attention spans in terms of nanoseconds when faced with the double whammy of estrogen overload and lack of sleep. So wading through the smart, but long, green solutions out there can land you somewhere between "maybe later" and, well, "never." If that sounds like you, you are going to love Ideal Bite! With a daily dose of green sense delivered right to your in-box, you can make positive changes without having a degree in environmental engineering . . . plus it's free!

"I was working seventy hours a week and had a full bank account but an empty emotional account. The whole corporate world is based on profit. I wanted to base a business on the profit of preservation. Then the dot-com crash happened; I was actually relieved and I took that as an opportunity to punch out. I went to Ireland and rode horses and thought for about a year. When I came back, I got a green MBA from George Washington University because I wanted to find a home, to do something aligned with my values and environmental passion.

"I started a consultancy business with Heather Stephenson (now my Ideal Bite partner) that helped companies figure out how to be more planet-friendly, how to go green. At the same time our friends were constantly asking us for advice: 'If I can't afford a Prius, what can I do to shrink my carbon footprint?' 'Can I be a vegetarian and still wear leather?' Well, we thought, why don't we invite all these green people over and get something going? That was the birth of Ideal Bite, bite-sized tidbits that are really doable. So maybe you're not perfect—that's all right, we're not, either. But what if you could find eco-friendly dog biscuits for your furry friend, or mailing boxes made out of recycled cardboard? Why not? It's a great place to start!"

Green Guru

Graham Hill
FOUNDER, TREEHUGGER.COM

This is a really comprehensive and lush-looking site with tons of information on the good green stuff you may want to surround yourself with. They're a little light on baby-specific gear, but there are enough ways to connect with folks there that—who knows?—you may want to start your own parenting group on Treehugger.

"When you have a child, you need so much stuff, and the consumer impact is huge. Now, I come from hippie parents, so the environmental movement is a natural for me. But it's important to be pragmatic. Hippies are a very small segment of society; in order for green to get big, we'd need to work *with* nature, not against it—human nature, I mean. People, including me, really like our 'stuff.' We care a lot about our homes, our cars, even our shampoos. We don't need to give these things up, but we may want to change how we look at them, and what we consider valuable. If we're going to be buying and using things, I want to make it easier, and more attractive, to go green.

"My idea was to create a vision of a green future that's meaningful, cool, and modern. Treehugger presents things that are green but that have an aesthetic that appeals to ninety-five percent of the population. We have 1,400,000 visitors a month, so this is not a fringe movement.

"People are very busy. It's not so easy to always do the right thing, especially when you have a little one. But if you could see all the beautiful green stuff in one place, it becomes possible to make the educated choices."

Green Guru

Chip Giller
FOUNDER, GRIST.ORG
NEW DAD

Grist is the real deal, the origin of the online green species. Perusing the "Ask Umbra" archives is like getting a degree in sustainability, but from a clever and funny professor. Witty and smart, this site reminded me that (a) I personally could make a huge difference, and (b) I do actually still have a brain and still have the ability to laugh at things other than my kids showing me their cute new made-up dances!

"We started a small newsletter and in four years it's just exploded. So we started Grist.org to be a gathering place for the next generation of environmentalists. They know that what happens on the planet now will affect them for a long time. This generation can lead our society into long-term change.

"We're at a point where we need green to become the norm, to be second nature, the lens through which all things are measured. Awareness is the first step. I have a thirteen-month-old daughter, and maybe it is a coincidence that I have seen so many positive changes in society since she was born, or maybe it's because your viewpoint changes so much when you are a parent—you see the good.

"People want to connect. To help each other. We hear from hundreds of readers each day, readers who talk to each other to share strategies on everything from green baby showers to nontoxic cleaners. Being a parent is really an opportunity to lead by example. Set a living model for your child, instill values.

"What can you do? There's a whole world out there to share ideas with. This is our time and our opportunity to make a difference. Our choices matter."

Green Flag
Some favorite sites for lactation support:

www.lalecheleague.org
www.breastfeeding.com
www.thebestfedbaby.com
www.militantbreastfeedingcult.com (not as weird as it sounds!)

For new-mom support:

www.cafemom.com (join a moms' group, or start your own—a bunch of green moms already did!)
www.parenting.ivillage.com (they've got a *lot* of great stuff goin' on over here; not too green, though—come on, let's convert some folks!)

For working moms online:

www.bluesuitmom.com

And that's just the beginning. There are so many more Web sites tailored precisely to *your* wants and needs. I have to be honest with you here: I am not the surfin' queen of the Internet. You're probably far more adept than me and can yell "Cowabunga!" and dive right in. But if you're feeling technically challenged (like me), remember, your trusty search engine knows what you're looking for! With a simple type and click you're ridin' the wave, and meeting and greeting new friends. . . .

YOUR BABY'S HEALTH CARE

No matter how green you are, and how healthy your baby is, you're going to need a baby doc, a pediatrician. You're probably not looking for an old-school type who knows it "all" but chooses to tell you very little (so as not to addle your girl brain). Your baby's doc doesn't have to be twinsies with your progressive way of thought, though. Choose someone who shares your feelings on breast-feeding, organic foods, etc., and who won't talk down to you just because of all that money and time in med school. On the other hand, don't expect a health-food co-op. Doctors may need to have antibacterials in the bathroom, but overall they can still be proponents of a healthy environment.

JUST WHAT THE DOCTOR ORDERED Here's what Lori Fraiser, a pediatrician in Salt Lake City, had to say: "There is a strong movement in medicine to avoid unnecessary antibiotics and also certain over-the-counter medications in younger age groups, but not all doctors are 'with the program.' I remember a mother yelling that she was going to spread the word we were a bad clinic because I would not give her kids antibiotics when they only had colds, and they were recovering, at that! She immediately went to another urgent clinic and got exactly what she wanted—antibiotics.

"Unfortunately, it's easier and quicker for the doctor to (inappropriately) prescribe antibiotics than explain why not and teach parents the signs to watch for that indicate they need to come back. Another contributing factor is that often both parents work, and not all employers are understanding about having a sick child. So the parents want the quick fix, not the careful observation, even though the quick fix doesn't work any better, and in fact it's worse in the long run.

"Don't get me wrong—antibiotics are invaluable and there's such a thing as going too far in the other direction. I know a case of a ten-year-old who died of a totally treatable form of meningitis when just a simple course of antibiotics would have saved her life. Essential oils and prayer were her treatment, because they were natural—but they weren't necessarily better."

THE TOUGHEST JOB YOU'LL EVER LOVE

There's a quote I often think of in regard to parenthood that for a long time I thought was said by some great statesman (Ben Franklin or Abe Lincoln, perhaps?). I often repeat it to myself: "With great power comes great responsibility." (Later I found out it was actually said to Peter Parker, aka Spider-Man, by his wise uncle, and that made me feel a little foolish. But anyway, great line, and deep meaning—thanks, Stan Lee!)

Or as our Green Guru Professor Marie Myung-Ok Lee puts it, "When I had my baby, it was daunting and awesome to find myself wholly responsible for the well-being of another person. I read a lot about mothering, but I also trusted the authorities. I assumed the doctors were keeping an eye on how much mercury my baby was getting in his vaccines, and that the government agencies were taking note of how much lead was in Christmas lights, lunch boxes, candles, and such. But now I know this: No one is really watching over your baby but YOU."

So what are your responsibilities, parentwise? These seem to change dramatically with every generation. Used to be your job included delivering harsh punishments and hard spankings at the least sign of insubordination. Other times it meant being sure your daughter knew how to cook and clean well enough to get and keep her man. Then there was the somewhat more reasonable and still important one of making enough dough to feed and clothe the little ones. But I'd like to say that now, in this generation, we have another great power, and great responsibility. Now more than ever, when TVs and Nintendos will soon enough try to usurp our draw, we must own our terrific bossiness. Not about bedtime or picking up toys (good luck with those), but about being the best "things" in our kids' lives, the real deal, the one authority.

MOTHERLAND: A PLACE WHERE EVERYTHING IS GOOD FOR BABY

Developmental psychologist Dr. Lisa Ecklund-Flores says it all: "Natural is better." Throughout this book I have tried to explain why natural is better. Thus far, "natural" has meant organic foods, scents, building materials, and clothing. Well, natural is better when it comes to child development, too.

"You are your child's connection, classroom, and museum," says Dr. Ecklund-Flores. "With Mom's and Dad's faces come their smells, their touch, and their voices—these are all natural, 'organic' sources of sensory stimulation that are crucial to normal development. It's time to stand firm with your natural instincts about what is important for your baby. It's time to recognize the importance of your role in your baby's development, because the most important, pervasive, and effective source of stimulation for your baby is YOU."

As I learned from Dr. Ecklund-Flores, early-childhood-development research tells us how a natural, "organic" approach to parenting is best for our babies.

• A newborn baby prefers her mother's voice, or any female voice, over any other sound.

Sage Moms: Talk to your baby! It's important for the development of memory, language, and emotional attachment.

• Touch is crucial to improve sleep and relaxation, reduce crying, and control stress hormones in newborn infants.

Sage Moms: Touch your baby! Infant massage and swaddling in baby slings are important sources of physical and emotional wellness.

• Infants and young children learn through physical exploration of the natural environment.

Sage Moms: Your baby will learn more effectively if you let him actively explore (anything!) than if you sit him in front of a computer or television.

- Unstructured, independent play is the most important source of stimulation for cognitive, emotional, and physical development in early childhood.

   Sage Moms: You don't need to rush your toddler to trendy classes every minute of every day—just give her time for open-ended play!

THIS LAND IS YOUR LAND

Everything you've ever dreamed of is imprinted in you and is possible for your baby: He is a shining example of newness. She is an open book, expecting fresh air, clean water, pure food, and an equal playing field. The conscious choices that you make create change. What would the world be like if every mother you knew committed to taking one of these small steps every day?

- Taking a walk

- Planting a tree

- Turning off the air conditioner

- Turning down the heat

- Eating dinner by candlelight

- Carrying reusable shopping bags

- Giving organic flowers

- Asking the grocery store to carry more organic goods

- Buying only local and in-season produce

You make the choices that form our world today and our children's world tomorrow.

Green Guru

Karenna Gore
MOTHER

For most of us, our green light will turn on when we become mothers. Part of our biological heritage of caring for our young is to be sure their environment is safe, from predators, poisons, threats of any kind. Here Karenna eloquently sums up the great siren call that's beating in our hearts and moving us all forward to a better way. (She comes by it quite naturally; her dad is Al Gore.)

"There is nothing as powerful as those innocent, vulnerable little eyes to remind us of the majesty of our charge to take care of the earth. Politicians often talk about 'future generations' in a vague way, but here they are, giggling, wondering, spilling milk on the rug, and you have to stop and think what kind of air, water, and land we will leave them to grow old in. I think the example parents set is as important as anything—picking up litter and throwing it away, recycling, speaking with respect for the farmers who make the fresh foods that go on the table—all these things send powerful messages to children about our place in the world. Every day mothers take care to protect their children from harmful foods, toxic cleaners, harsh rays of the sun—the earth itself needs that kind of love, and mothers can lead the way in giving it."

The end of my book is just the beginning of your journey. I want to thank you for including me in this wonderful time in your life. I hope you've found some ideas and insights to make your most important job a little easier. And I wanted to mention something you already know:

You are the luckiest person in the world, having that wonderful baby.

And you are also one of the most powerful.

The hand that rocks the cradle rules the world. The choices you make today are ones your child will live with for many tomorrows.

Enjoy your journey. I guarantee you'll love it. This is the one job that you'll be happy never ends.

You'll be a mother for the rest of your life.

GREEN AT A GLANCE

Evergreen: Make a commitment to yourself to surround yourself with people who support your sustainable world view. (Even if they are virtual friends.)

Pea green: Take baby steps into a kinder environment. Walk to the park instead of driving. Stop by the weekend farmers' market for tonight's salad.

Spring green: Whether you are working or not, be sure to carve out bonding time between you and baby. Kick back and goof off with baby. Take a walk with him or take a nap with her. Being together will strengthen your confidence in your decisions and instill in you the leadership qualities you'll need as a mom.

Green Goods

How to find out more about some of the great people and organizations you read about in the book, as well as others that I hope you will find useful . . .

One

Blue Hill at Stone Barns
Organic and local restaurant
630 Bedford Rd
Pocantico Hills, NY 10591
(914) 366-9600
www.bluehillstonebarns.com

Coffee Labs Roasters
Certified organic coffee roaster
7 Main Street
Tarrytown, NY 10591
(914) 332-1479

Organic Trade Association
Nonprofit that is the heart of the organic movement

PO Box 547
Greenfield, MA 01302
(413) 774-7511
www.ota.com

Waterkeeper Alliance
Worldwide nonprofit working to protect our water from pollution
50 S. Buckhout, Suite 302
Irvington, NY 10533
(914) 674-0622
www.waterkeeper.org

Organic and natural food stores, farms, and manufacturers

Amy's Kitchen
www.amys.com

Annie's Naturals
www.consorzio.com

Earth's Best
www.earthsbest.com

Organic Valley Family of Farms
www.organicvalley.coop

Seeds of Change
www.seedsofchange.com

Stonyfield Farm
www.stonyfield.com

Whole Foods Market
www.wholefoods.com

Two

Dr. Hauschka
The finest biodynamic and organic skin care
59 North Street
Hatfield, MA 01038
(800) 247-9907
www.drhauschka.com

The Campaign for Safe Cosmetics
Comprehensive information and campaigns for safer cosmetics, focusing on phthalates
www.safecosmetics.org

Environmental Working Group
Industry-leading nonprofit with searchable database that allows you to track toxicity levels of thousands of name-brand cosmetics
1436 U Street NW, Suite 100
Washington, DC 20009
(202) 667-6982
www.ewg.org

Karim Orange
Makeup artist and natural-cosmetic expert
www.karimorange.com

MyChelle
A great line of very "clean" and natural makeup that's accessibly priced
www.mychelleusa.com

Three

Firozé
Clean products and treatment line from the industry expert
www.firoze.com

John Masters Organics
Salon
www.johnmasters.com
77 Sullivan Street
New York, NY 10012
(212) 343-9590
Hair and beauty products
(800) 599-2450

Locks of Love
Nonprofit that takes shorn human hair and turns it into hairpieces for people in need (check this out, you'll be amazed!)
www.locksoflove.org

Pangea
Super green and clean body care and hair care products
pangeaorganics.com

Peacekeeper
Formaldehyde-free nail polish—all profits benefit human rights
www.iamapeacekeeper.com

Priti Organic Spa
One of the greatest experiences your feet will ever have, and toxin-free!
35 East First Street

New York, NY 10003
(212) 254-3628
www.pritiorganicspa.com

Four

Bluecorn Naturals
Beautiful nontoxic candles
www.beeswaxcandles.com

Kuumba Made
Handmade coconut oil salves and fragrances
www.kuumbamade.com

U.S. Environmental Protection Agency
Ariel Rios Building
1200 Pennsylvania Avenue NW
Washington, DC 20460
www.cpa.gov

Weleda
Some of the finest organic and biodynamic body care and baby body care on the market
1 Closter Road
PO Box 675
Palisades, NY 10964
(800) 241-1030
www.usa.weleda.com

Five

Farmer Steve's Popcorn
Such fine popcorn, and not genetically modified!
www.farmersteve.com

Garden of Eatin'
Great to pig out on if you want something that tastes junky but is actually natural. Available tons of places—key in to store locator to see where.
gardenofeatin.com

Green Field Paper Company
The best selection of handmade paper—including the superfun Grow-A-Note, which you can plant after use!
www.greenfieldpaper.com

It's Only Natural
One of the first organic-only clothing and gift stores. Big selection of women's and babies' organic cotton.
407 West Gregory
Kansas City, MO 64114
(816) 523-7434
www.itsonlynatural.us

Newman's Own
Yummy, natural, and/or organic—plus, all the after-tax proceeds go to charity!
www.newmansown.com

Recycled Paper Greetings
Great recycled cards
www.recycledpapergreetings.com

The Rooster Crows
Really beautiful cards for every occasion
www.theroostercrows.com

Walnut Acres
Probably the oldest, and certainly one of the finest, in mail-order organics
www.walnutacres.com

World of Good
The most beautiful handmade crafts and gifts ever! Traded fairly and made with artisans in women's cooperatives around the world.
www.worldofgood.com

Six

BabyGanics
Superclean cleaning products that are totally safe for baby. The lavender scent is so soothing!
www.babyganics.com

Deirdre Imus
Information on the Deirdre Imus Environmental Center for Pediatric Oncology and links to her green cleaning book
www.dienviro.com

Seventh Generation
The pioneer in green clean—plus great recycled paper products.
www.seventhgeneration.com

Seven

Burt's Bees
Accessibly priced natural body care. Available nationwide, too.
www.burtsbees.com

Naturepedic
The finest baby mattresses on the planet
www.naturepedic.com

New Native Inc.
The mother of all baby slings
www.newnativeinc.com

Eight

Environmental Justice Foundation
Get ready for this hard-hitting, unforgettable UK nonprofit, and the better world they are striving for.
www.ejfoundation.org

gDiapers
Disposable inserts in cloth covers
www.gdiapers.com

Pesticide Action Network North America
"Advancing alternatives to pesticides worldwide"
www.panna.org

Texas Organic Cotton Marketing Cooperative
*The farmers' cooperative I first read about, which inspired me to start
Green Babies. Cliff Bingham is a member.*
www.texasorganic.com

Tiny Tush
Every possible kind of cloth diaper
www.tinytush.com

Tushies
Dioxin- and gel-free disposables
www.tushies.com

More Cloth Diapers

Baby Bunz & Co.
www.babybunz.com

Green Mountain Diapers
www.greenmountaindiapers.com

Katie's Kisses
www.katieskisses.com

Nine

Kids for Saving Earth
*Fun stuff to turn kids green; nonprofit educational material
for all ages*
KSE Worldwide
PO Box 421118
Minneapolis, MN 55442

(763) 559-1234
www.kidsforsavingearth.org

Green Fertility
Thoughtful and sometimes hilarious essays on parenting and life
greenfertility.blogspot.com

Green Nest
Everything you need appliance-wise to clean up your home act eco-wise, from a couple who are really knowledgeable
www.greennest.com

Healthy Child Healthy World
An easy-to-navigate terrific go-to on children's toxicity issues
www.healthychild.org

IKEA
The Swedish home-furnishings giant has a very clean outlook, using nonthreatened hardwoods and banning the most toxic flame retardants in their mattresses and sofas.
www.ikea.com

Q Collection
Furniture for Junior and you, crafted in the U.S. from sustainably harvested wood
www.qcollection.com

Vivavi
Fantastic collection of green home furnishings
www.vivavi.com

Ten

BornFree
Safe baby bottles and sippy cups
www.newbornfree.com

The Future of Food
Fascinating movie from Deborah Koons Garcia on the drama and dangers of genetically modified food
www.thefutureoffood.com

Mothers & Menus
Delivery—what a relief!
In NYC: (646) 522-9591
www.mothersandmenus.com

The Organic Center
Nonprofit formed to "generate credible, peer-reviewed scientific information and communicate the verifiable benefits of organic farming and products to society"
www.organiccenter.org

Eleven

Beyond Pesticides
Nonprofit. The most comprehensive site on the dangers of pesticides, civil action against them, and doable steps you can take to lessen your exposure.
701 E Street SE, Suite 200
Washington, DC 20003
(202) 543-5450
www.beyondpesticides.org

NaturaLawn of America
Organic-based lawn care
www.nl-amer.com

Our Children's Toxic Legacy: How Science and Law Fail to Protect Us from Pesticides
Book by John Wargo
yalepress.yale.edu/yupbooks/book.asp?isbn=9780300074468

Pesticide Action Network of North America (PANNA)
Another terrific and informative nonprofit
www.panna.org

Twelve

Earth's Best
The mother of all organic baby food. Available oodles of places, or order online.
www.earthsbest.com

Fresh Baby
These generous sisters will teach you everything you need to know about making and freezing your own baby food. Terrific kit has whatever you need. Available at Whole Foods and Babies "R" Us.
616 Petoskey Street, Suite 202
Petoskey, MI 49770
(231) 348-2706
www.freshbaby.com

Fresh Daisy Organic
As far as I know, the original frozen organic baby food. Wide

availability in the UK. A passionate pioneer and advocate for children's health.
www.daisyfoods.com

Happy Baby
Super-yummy gourmet frozen baby food
www.happybabyfood.com

Nice Cubes
Frozen cubes of organic baby food
www.nicecubesbaby.com

Plum Organics
More convenient organic frozen baby food
www.plumorganics.com

Vegetarian Baby & Child
Online magazine offering advice on raising vegetarian and vegan babies up to teens. Recipes, nutrition, health information, and veggie articles.
www.vegetarianbaby.com

Vegetarian Times
Magazine. Offers tips and recipes on simple, delicious food that is strictly vegetarian.
www.vegetariantimes.com

Thirteen

Body & Soul
Magazine. Martha's marvelous take on whole living.
www.bodyandsoulmag.com

Co-op America

A nonprofit that has been around forever (about as long as my business!) working to connect consumers to clean, green, and ethical businesses. Membership has a bunch of perks.
www.coopamerica.org

E

The most informative and yet readable magazine on green ever. A great gift to yourself.
www.emagazine.com

Fit Pregnancy

Magazine. Very green but also keeps you looking snazzy. Not just for pregnancy—lots for new moms, too.
www.fitpregnancy.com

Grist

Love this green site. It's original and very witty—made me feel like a smartie, and after I surfed it a bit, indeed I was!
www.grist.org

Ideal Bite

Fun daily green tips to your e-mail
www.idealbite.com

An Inconvenient Truth

Movie. Al Gore's comprehensible yet dramatic exploration of the issue of our time, global warming, and how we can take back our power and stop it.
www.climatecrisis.net

Laurie David
This passionate and beautiful activist is the real reason most of us even know what global warming is. Her book, Stop Global Warming: The Solution Is You, *may be a survival guide for our species.*
www.lauriedavid.com

Mothering
The real deal on a totally natural approach. The mother of all mothering mags.
www.mothering.com

National Resources Defense Council
One of the nation's most powerful environmental groups
40 West Twentieth Street
New York, NY 10011
(212) 727-2700
www.nrdc.org

Plenty
A fun, fashionable green mag, great looking.
www.plentymag.com

Prenatal Yoga Center
Terrifically helpful site. You can ask questions of an array of experts.
251 West Seventy-second Street 2F
New York, NY
(212) 362-2985
www.prenatalyogacenter.com

Real Simple
Magazine. Gorgeous and natural; lots of doable how-tos on a greener, better lifestyle.
www.realsimple.com

Stop Global Warming

Fun and comprehensive site on grassroots movements and day-to-day tips to make the little changes that result in big differences. Even if you can't leave your house, you can join a virtual march. This site is not a downer—check it out.

www.stopglobalwarming.org

TreeHugger

Well-researched, vast site. Like having a chic, smart, green personal shopper.

www.treehugger.com

Photo Credits

Part One: Linda Skoog
Chapter One: Linda Skoog
Chapter Two: H. Fassa
Chapter Three: Linda Skoog
Chapter Four: H. Fassa
Chapter Five: Linda Skoog
Chapter Six: Linda Skoog
Part Two: Linda Skoog
Chapter Seven: Linda Skoog
Chapter Eight: Linda Skoog
Chapter Nine: Linda Skoog
Chapter Ten: Linda Skoog
Part Three: Linda Skoog
Chapter Eleven: H. Fassa
Chapter Twelve: Linda Skoog
Chapter Thirteen: Linda Skoog